GoodFood

101 MORE LOW-FAT FEASTS

10 9 8 7 6 5 4 3 2 1

Published in 2010 by BBC Books, an imprint of
Ebury Publishing
A Random House Group company

Recipes © BBC Magazines 2010
Book design © Woodlands Books Ltd 2010
All photographs © BBC Magazines 2010
All recipes contained within this book first appeared in
BBC *Good Food* magazine.

The Random House Group Limited Reg. No. 954009

Addresses for companies within the Random House
Group can be found at www.randomhouse.co.uk

A CIP catalogue record for this book is available from
the British Library.

The Random House Group Limited supports The
Forest Stewardship Council (FSC), the leading
international forest certification organization. All our
titles that are printed on Greenpeace approved
FSC certified paper carry the FSC logo. Our paper
procurement policy can be found at www.rbooks.
co.uk/environment

Printed and bound by Firmengruppe APPL, aprinta
druck, Wemding, Germany
Colour origination by Dot Gradations Ltd, UK

Commissioning Editor: Muna Reyal
Project Editor: Joe Cottington
Designer: Annette Peppis
Production: David Brimble
Picture Researcher: Gabby Harrington

ISBN: 9781846079146

To buy books by your favourite authors and register for
offers visit www.rbooks.co.uk

Picture and recipe credits

BBC *Good Food* magazine and BBC Books would
like to thank the following people for providing photos.
While every effort has been made to trace and
acknowledge all photographers, we should like to
apologize should there be any errors or omissions.

Steve Baxter p137, p167; Peter Cassidy p73, p169,
p203; Jean Cazals p79, p181; Dean Grennan p67,
p157; Will Heap p29, p109, p163; Gareth Morgans
p21, p25, p31, p41, p49, p63, p69, p75, p87, p155,
p179; David Munns p19, p33, p39, p43, p47, p61,
p99, p107, p125, p159, p171, p173, p183, p185,
p193; Myles New p13, p15, p11, p23, p35, p37,
p45, p51, p53, p65, p71, p77, p81, p83, p85, p93,
p101, p103, p111, p141, p145, p149, p151, p201;
Lis Parsons p27, p113, p115, p139, p197; Craig
Robertson p55, p59, p105, p121, p129, p135, p153,
p191, p205, p209; Howard Shooter p123, p165;
Brett Stevens p117; Roger Stowell p17, p131, p161,
p187, p195, p199; Simon Walton p57, p147, p177,
p207; Philip Webb p89, p91, p95, p97, p119, p189,
p211; Simon Wheeler p127, p133, p175

All the recipes in this book were created by
the editorial team at *Good Food* and by regular
contributors to the magazine.

For 6,000 recipes you can trust see bbcgoodfood.com

GoodFood

101 MORE LOW-FAT FEASTS
TRIPLE-TESTED RECIPES

Editor
Sharon Brown

BOOKS

Contents

Introduction   6

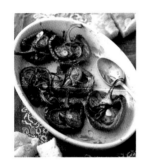 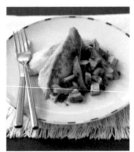 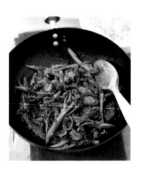

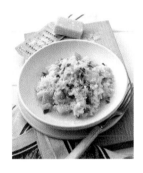
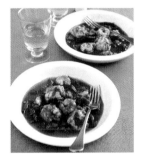
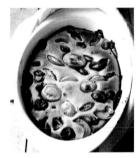

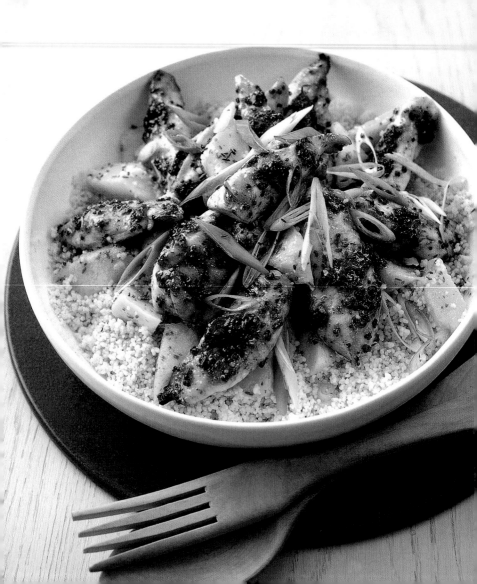

Introduction

Low in fat but packed with flavour – that's the theme of the recipes in this book. Getting a good balance of foods in our everyday eating is the answer to a healthy diet, and choosing low-fat dishes within your weekly menus is a good starting point.

How you cook is as important as what you cook: low-fat methods of cooking include grilling and griddling, as both of these allow the fat simply to drain away. Steaming veg is a good way to retain the nutrients and vibrant colour, and stir-frying is good too, as you only need a little oil. With this collection, we've taken 101 of *Good Food* magazine's favourite recipes, complete with all sorts of different cooking techniques, so you'll never have to suffer a dull, lifeless low-fat meal again!

We've included one-pots (they're simple to cook and save on the washing up), fast suppers (all cooked and on the table in 30 minutes), a selection of weekend specials for when you have a little more time, delicious vegetarian ideas and some irresistible guilt-free puds – and all low in fat. As with all *Good Food* recipes, these have been tried and triple-tested in our kitchen, so delicious results are guaranteed!

Sharon

Sharon Brown
Good Food magazine

Notes and conversion tables

NOTES ON THE RECIPES
• Eggs are large in the UK and Australia and extra large in America unless stated otherwise.
• Wash fresh produce before preparation.
• Recipes contain nutritional analyses for 'sugar', which means the total sugar content including all natural sugars in the ingredients, unless otherwise stated.

OVEN TEMPERATURES

Gas	°C	°C Fan	°F	Oven temp.
¼	110	90	225	Very cool
½	120	100	250	Very cool
1	140	120	275	Cool or slow
2	150	130	300	Cool or slow
3	160	140	325	Warm
4	180	160	350	Moderate
5	190	170	375	Moderately hot
6	200	180	400	Fairly hot
7	220	200	425	Hot
8	230	210	450	Very hot
9	240	220	475	Very hot

APPROXIMATE WEIGHT CONVERSIONS
• All the recipes in this book list both imperial and metric measurements. Conversions are approximate and have been rounded up or down. Follow one set of measurements only; do not mix the two.
• Cup measurements, which are used by cooks in Australia and America, have not been listed here as they vary from ingredient to ingredient. Kitchen scales should be used to measure dry/solid ingredients.

Good Food are concerned about sustainable sourcing and animal welfare so where possible, we use organic ingredients, humanely-reared meats, free-range chickens and eggs and unrefined sugar.

SPOON MEASURES

Spoon measurements are level unless otherwise specified.

- 1 teaspoon (tsp) = 5ml
- 1 tablespoon (tbsp) = 15ml
- 1 Australian tablespoon = 20ml (cooks in Australia should measure 3 teaspoons where 1 tablespoon is specified in a recipe)

APPROXIMATE LIQUID CONVERSIONS

metric	imperial	AUS	US
50ml	2fl oz	¼ cup	¼ cup
125ml	4fl oz	½ cup	½ cup
175ml	6fl oz	¾ cup	¾ cup
225ml	8fl oz	1 cup	1 cup
300ml	10fl oz/½ pint	½ pint	1¼ cups
450ml	16fl oz	2 cups	2 cups/1 pint
600ml	20fl oz/1 pint	1 pint	2½ cups
1 litre	35fl oz/1¾ pints	1¾ pints	1 quart

Trout is fabulous – it is an excellent source of those all-important omega-3 oils and contains just a third of the calories of salmon.

Smoked trout and cucumber open sandwiches

125g pack skinless hot-smoked trout fillets
½ × 250g tub Quark
½–1 tsp horseradish sauce
a squeeze of fresh lemon juice
2 thick slices granary bread
¼ cucumber, sliced
25g/1oz watercress
2 handfuls of cherry tomatoes, to serve

Takes 20 minutes • Serves 2

1 Flake the fish into a large bowl, then stir in the Quark and horseradish sauce to taste. Season with black pepper and a squeeze of lemon juice.
2 Toast the bread, then top each piece with cucumber slices and watercress. Spoon half the trout pâté on top of each and serve with halved cherry tomatoes on the side.

• Per serving 268 kcalories, protein 29g, carbohydrate 25g, fat 7g, saturated fat 2g, fibre 3g, sugar 5g, salt 1.3g

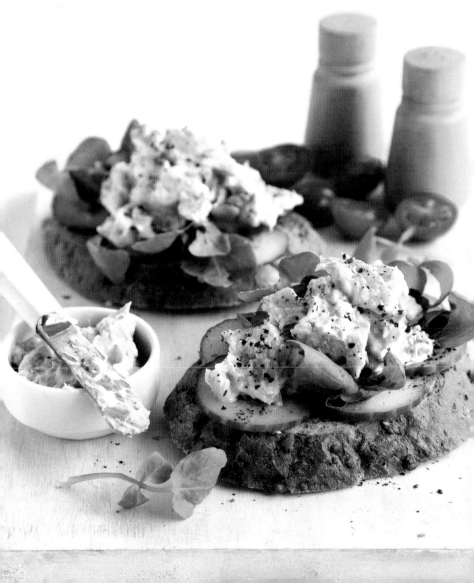

The aromatic Asian-style sesame, lime and ginger dressing in this recipe goes brilliantly with pasta, which is, after all, the European equivalent of the noodle.

Superfood pasta salad

300g/10oz wholewheat penne
250g/9oz frozen soya beans
250g pack green beans,
trimmed and halved
1 tsp sesame oil
1 tbsp soy sauce
small knob of ginger, grated
juice of 1 lime
50g/2oz alfalfa sprouts or cress
2 carrots, grated
1 small bunch coriander, leaves
roughly chopped

Takes 20 minutes • Serves 4

1 Cook the pasta according to the packet instructions, adding the soya beans and green beans 3 minutes before the end of cooking. Drain, tip into a colander, then cool quickly under cold running water.
2 Whisk together the oil, soy sauce, ginger and lime juice in a large bowl, then tip in the pasta, cooked beans, alfalfa sprouts or cress, carrots and coriander. Toss the salad well, then serve.

• Per serving 379 kcalories, protein 20g, carbohydrate 63g, fat 7g, saturated fat 1g, fibre 12g, sugar 8g, salt 0.96g

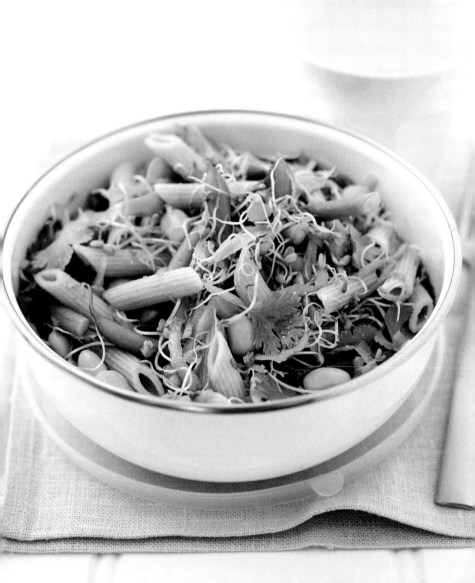

These full-of-flavour peppers make a great low-fat side dish with just about anything, or serve them on their own with chunks of bread.

Roasted peppers with tomatoes and anchovies

4 red peppers, halved and seeded
50g can anchovies in oil, drained
and oil reserved
8 smallish tomatoes, halved
2 garlic cloves, thinly sliced
2 rosemary sprigs
2 tbsp olive oil
bread or focaccia, to serve

Takes 1 hour 20 minutes • Serves 4

1 Preheat the oven to 160°C/140°C fan/ gas 3. Put the peppers into a large baking dish, toss with a little of the oil from the anchovy can, then turn cut-side up. Roast for 40 minutes, until soft but not collapsed.
2 Slice 8 of the anchovies along their length. Put 2 halves of tomato, several garlic slices, a few little rosemary sprigs and 2 pieces of anchovy into the hollow of each pepper. Drizzle over the olive oil, then roast again for 30 minutes until the tomatoes are soft and the peppers are filled with pools of tasty juice. Leave to cool and serve warm or at room temperature, with some bread or focaccia on the side, if you like.

• Per serving 162 kcalories, protein 4g, carbohydrate 13g, fat 11g, saturated fat 1g, fibre 3g, sugar 12g, salt 1.44g

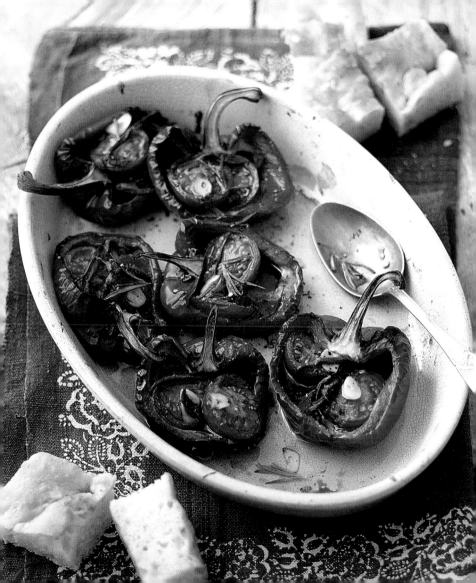

This healthy, fill-you-up soup contains five of your 5-a-day in one bowl. You can use whatever vegetables are in season – just choose your favourites. Delicious served with granary bread.

Cauliflower, pumpkin and bean soup

1 tbsp olive oil
2 onions, chopped
2 garlic cloves, chopped
500g/1lb 2oz pumpkin or squash, peeled, seeded and chopped
1 potato, chopped
several thyme sprigs, leaves stripped
1 litre/1¾ pints vegetable stock
500g/1lb 2oz cauliflower, cut into small florets
400g can haricot beans, drained and rinsed
a handful of chopped parsley
crusty bread, to serve

Takes 55 minutes • Serves 4

1 Heat the oil in a large pan, add the onions, then fry for about 10 minutes until soft and lightly coloured. Stir in the garlic, pumpkin or squash, potato and thyme, then cook for 1 minute.
2 Pour in the stock, then bring to the boil. Reduce the heat, cover, simmer for around 20 minutes, then add the cauliflower and beans, and cook for a further 10 minutes until all the vegetables are tender.
3 Remove about two ladlefuls of soup and pour into a food processor, then add the parsley and process until smooth – taking good care not to splash yourself with the hot liquid. Return to the pan, then reheat and serve with some crusty bread.

• Per serving 215 kcalories, protein 13g, carbohydrate 31g, fat 5g, saturated fat none, fibre 10g, sugar 12g, salt 1.01g

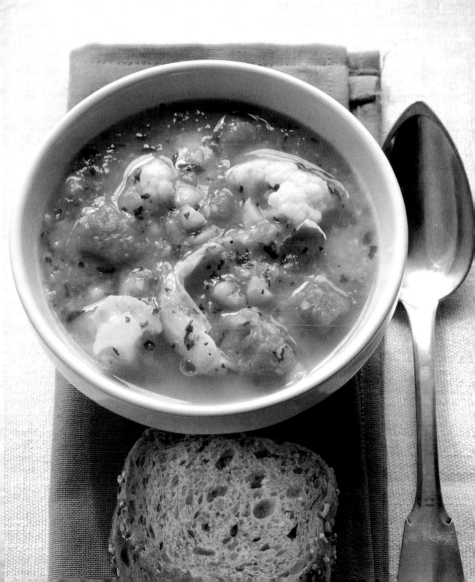

Quinoa is a wonderful ingredient and makes a great substitute for rice or couscous. It's a seed, not a grain, so it is an excellent source of protein and has a satisfying texture.

Quinoa, lentil and feta salad

200g/8oz quinoa
1 tsp olive oil
1 shallot or ½ onion, finely chopped
2 tbsp tarragon, roughly chopped
400g can Puy or green lentils, drained and rinsed
¼ cucumber, peeled and diced
100g/4oz feta, crumbled
6 spring onions, thinly sliced
zest and juice of 1 orange
1 tbsp red or white wine vinegar

Takes 30 minutes • Serves 4

1 Cook the quinoa in a large pan of boiling water for 10–15 minutes until tender, drain well, then set aside to cool.

2 Meanwhile, heat the oil in a small pan, then cook the shallot or onion for a few minutes until softened. Add the tarragon, stir well, then remove from the heat.

3 Stir the softened shallot and tarragon into the cooled quinoa along with the lentils, cucumber, feta, spring onions, orange zest and juice and vinegar. Toss well together and chill until ready to serve.

• Per serving 286 kcalories, protein 16g, carbohydrate 39g, fat 9g, saturated fat 3g, fibre 2g, sugar 6g, salt 1.48g

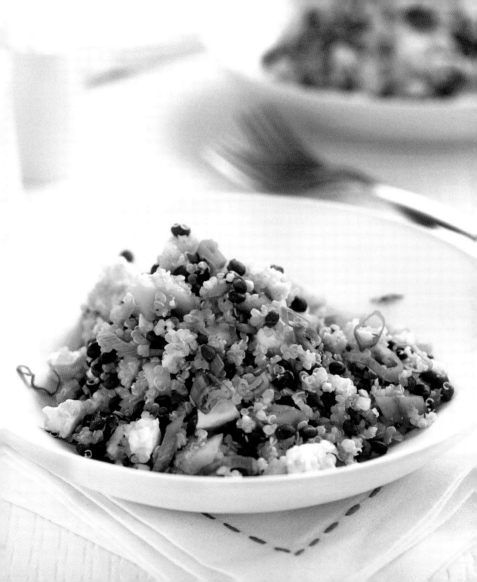

The flavourful Vietnamese-style dressing for this crunchy salad is best made just before serving to preserve the vibrant colour of the mint.

Crunchy prawn noodle salad

100g/4oz rice noodles
100g/4oz sugar snap peas, shredded
2 carrots, coarsely grated
100g/4oz baby leaf spinach
85g/3oz cooked peeled prawns
(defrosted if frozen)

FOR THE DRESSING
1 red chilli, seeded and
finely chopped
3 tbsp rice vinegar
1 tsp caster sugar
1 tsp fish sauce
1 tbsp roughly chopped mint

Takes 20 minutes • Serves 2

1 Pour boiling water over the noodles to cover, leave for 4 minutes, then cool under cold running water. Drain well.
2 Mix the sugar snaps, carrots, spinach, noodles and prawns in a shallow bowl. Mix together the dressing ingredients until the sugar has dissolved, pour over the salad, then toss everything together. Serve it up straight away.

• Per serving 278 kcalories, protein 15g, carbohydrate 55g, fat 1g, saturated fat none, fibre 4g, sugar 13g, salt 1.43g

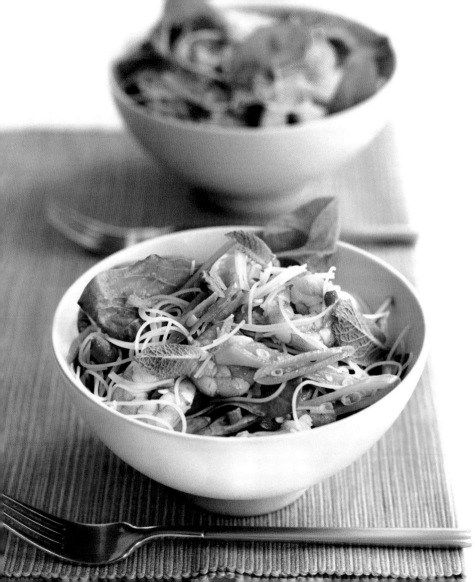

You can find Peppadew peppers in jars in most supermarkets.
Their lovely sweet-and-sour flavour works especially well on pizzas.
Serve these tasty low-fat snacks with a crisp green salad, if you like.

Ciabatta pizzas with sticky onions

1 tbsp olive oil
2 large onions, thinly sliced
1 garlic clove, sliced
leaves from 2 rosemary sprigs, chopped
10 Peppadew peppers from a jar, quartered
3 tbsp black olives, pitted and halved
1 ciabatta loaf, sliced lengthways and halved
2 handfuls of grated Gruyère or Cheddar

Takes 30 minutes • Serves 4

1 Preheat the oven to 200°C/180°C fan/ gas 6 and heat the oil in a large, lidded frying pan. Add the onions, garlic and rosemary with a splash of water, cover, then cook for about 10 minutes until soft. Remove the lid, turn up the heat, then cook the mixture for a few more minutes.

2 Stir in the peppers, olives and some seasoning. Put the ciabatta halves facing upwards on a baking sheet. Divide the mixture over the bread, spreading a little to cover. Sprinkle over the cheese, then bake for 10 minutes or until the cheese is bubbling.

• Per serving 357 kcalories, protein 13g, carbohydrate 51g, fat 12g, saturated fat 4g, fibre 4g, sugar 12g, salt 1.5g

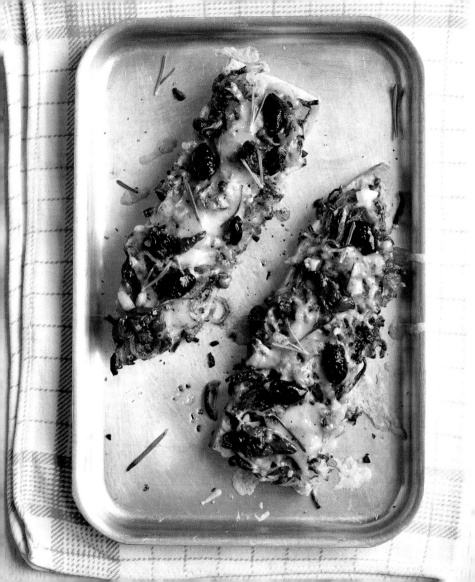

The ham and crispy bacon turn this deliciously thick soup into something a bit special. It's healthy too, as it is high in fibre and contains two of your 5-a-day.

Hearty Tuscan bean soup

2 tbsp olive oil, plus extra to drizzle
1 celery stick, chopped
1 onion, chopped
1 large carrot, chopped
700ml/1¼ pint stock
400g can cannellini beans in water, drained
400g can borlotti beans in water, drained
1 rosemary sprig
1 thyme sprig
1 bay leaf
140g/5oz cooked ham, shredded
8 prosciutto slices or streaky bacon rashers, fried or grilled, to garnish

Takes 30 minutes • Serves 4

1 Heat the oil in a large pan, then add the chopped vegetables and some salt and pepper. Cook very gently for 10 minutes until softened but not coloured.
2 Add the stock, beans, rosemary and thyme sprigs and the bay leaf. Bring to the boil, then simmer for 10 minutes.
3 Lift out the herbs then, using a stick blender, whiz to a roughly chunky but creamy soup. Stir in the ham and bring to a simmer. Serve garnished with a few crisp prosciutto slices or bacon rashers and a swirl of olive oil.

• Per serving 248 kcalories, protein 17g, carbohydrate 28g, fat 8g, saturated fat 1g, fibre 8g, sugar 8g, salt 1.33g

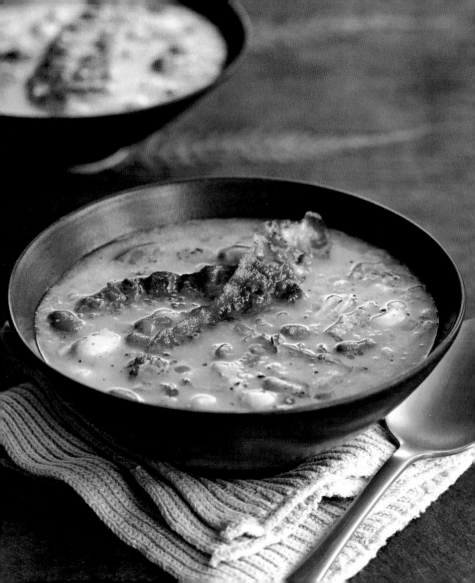

This fresh-tasting salad is perfect for making ahead, but take it out of the fridge a good hour before serving to allow the flavours to develop.

Lemony potato, broccoli and goat's cheese salad

500g bag new potatoes
1 tbsp extra-virgin olive oil
zest and juice of 1 lemon
1 broccoli head, cut into florets
200g/8oz green beans, trimmed
20g pack dill, leaves
roughly chopped
100g/4oz goat's cheese
2 tbsp toasted pine nuts

Takes 35 minutes, plus cooling
Serves 4

1 Boil the potatoes for 12–15 minutes until tender. Mix together the oil, lemon zest and juice in a serving bowl. Lift out the potatoes with a slotted spoon, leaving the pan of water on the hob. Drain the potatoes well, then place them in the serving bowl. Leave on one side to cool.
2 Add the broccoli and beans to the pan of boiling water. Cook for 4 minutes until tender but still with some bite. Drain, then cool under cold running water.
3 Stir the drained broccoli and beans into the cooled potatoes with the dill and some seasoning. Break the goat's cheese into chunks and scatter over the vegetables with the pine nuts and serve.

• Per serving 237 kcalories, protein 10g, carbohydrate 24g, fat 12g, saturated fat 3g, fibre 4g, sugar 4g, salt 0.35g

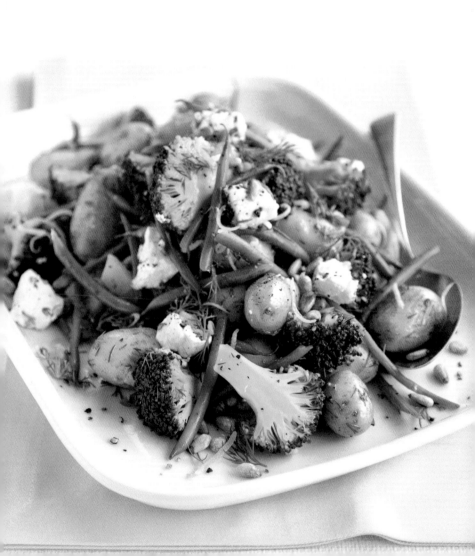

Served with pitta bread and tomato salsa, these meatballs make a great snack. You can use any kind of minced meat for this recipe, and the kids can help make them too.

Spicy meatballs

500g/1lb 2oz minced chicken, turkey, lamb, beef or pork
1 medium onion, chopped
2 garlic cloves, crushed or chopped
2 tsp mild or medium curry powder
2 tsp ground cumin
1 tsp garam masala
½ tsp paprika or cayenne pepper
2 tbsp chopped coriander
1 egg, beaten
50g/2oz fresh breadcrumbs
1 tbsp oil
crisp green salad, pitta bread and tomato salsa, to serve

Takes 40 minutes • Serves 6

1 Preheat the oven to 180°C/160°C fan/gas 4. Mix together the mince, onion, garlic, curry powder, cumin, garam masala, paprika or cayenne pepper and coriander. Add the beaten egg and breadcrumbs, then mix again. Divide the mixture into 18 even-sized pieces and shape into walnut-sized balls.
2 Heat the oil in a frying pan over a medium heat, add the meatballs and cook for around 5 minutes, turning until they are golden brown. Remove from the pan and place them on a baking sheet. Bake in the oven for 15–20 minutes.
3 Allow the meatballs to cool slightly and serve with a fresh, crisp green salad, some pitta bread and tomato salsa.

• Per serving 173 kcalories, protein 23g, carbohydrate 10g, fat 5g, saturated fat 1g, fibre 1g, sugar 1g, salt 0.35g

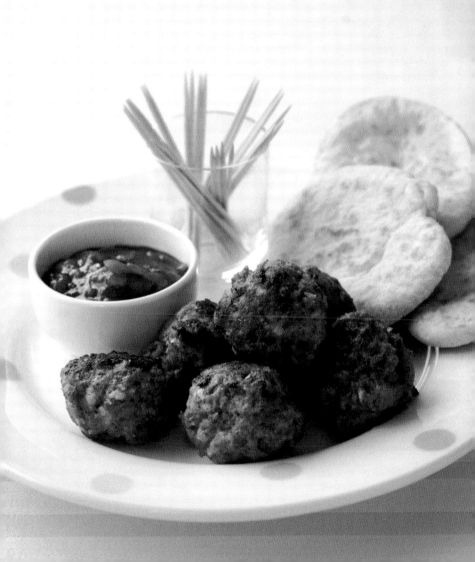

Nothing beats a bowl of warming home-made soup on a cold day to welcome home the family. This classic combination of flavours is always a winner.

Carrot and coriander soup

1 tbsp vegetable oil
1 onion, chopped
1 tsp ground coriander
1 potato, roughly chopped
450g/1lb carrots, chopped
1.2 litres/2 pints vegetable stock
1 × 28g pack coriander, leaves only

Takes 40 minutes • Serves 4

1 Heat the oil in a large pan, add the onion, then fry for 5 minutes until softened. Stir in the ground coriander and potato, then cook for 1 minute. Add the carrots and vegetable stock, bring to the boil, then reduce the heat. Cover and cook for 20 minutes until the carrots are tender.

2 Tip into a food processor with the coriander (reserving a few leaves for the garnish) then blitz until smooth – you may need to do this in two batches. Return to the pan, taste, and add seasoning if necessary. Reheat to serve, garnished with the remaining coriander leaves.

• Per serving 115 kcalories, protein 3g, carbohydrate 19g, fat 4g, saturated fat 1g, fibre 5g, sugar 12g, salt 0.46g

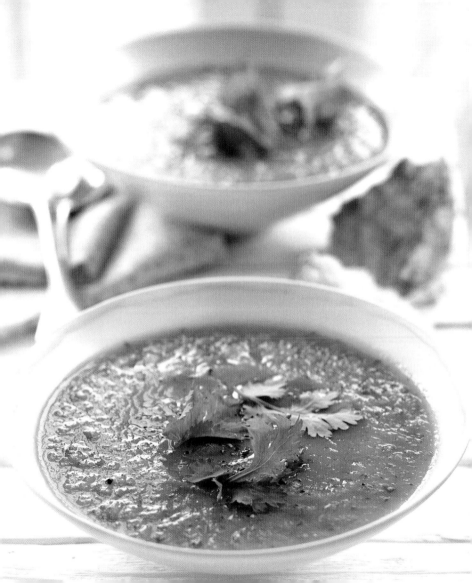

An easy-to-cook, healthy pizza-style dish topped with a peppery tomato salad makes a speedy and satisfying lunch that's on the table in 20 minutes.

Potato and chorizo pizza breads

3 medium to large potatoes, very thinly sliced
4 wholemeal tortillas
6 tbsp half-fat crème fraîche
½ onion, thinly sliced
8 thin slices chorizo from a pack, diced
25g/1oz mature Cheddar, grated
3 tomatoes, roughly chopped
2 tsp balsamic dressing
½ × 50g bag rocket leaves

Takes 20 minutes • Serves 4

1 Preheat the oven to 200°C/180°C fan/gas 6. Bring a pan of water to the boil, then blanch the potato slices in it for 2 minutes until almost cooked. Drain well, then tip on to kitchen paper to dry.
2 Put the tortillas on to baking sheets. Season the crème fraîche, then spread over the tortillas. Top with the potato slices, onion and chorizo, then scatter over the grated cheese. Bake for 8 minutes until golden.
3 Meanwhile, mix the tomatoes with the dressing and ½ teaspoon coarsely ground black pepper, then toss through the rocket.
4 Pile a quarter of the salad in the middle of each cooked tortilla and serve.

• Per serving 287 kcalories, protein 11g, carbohydrate 37g, fat 12g, saturated fat 5g, fibre 5g, sugar 5g, salt 1.01g

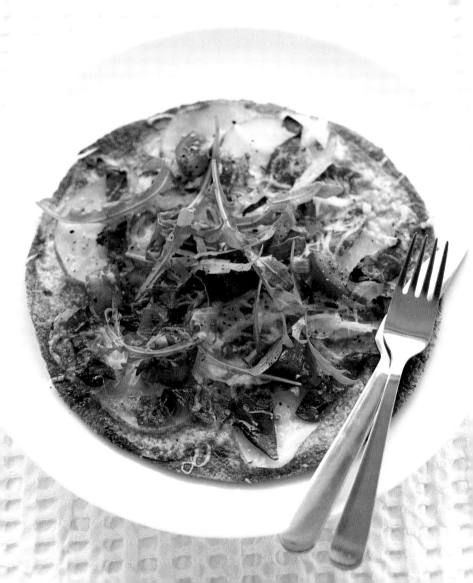

If you don't want to buy ready-prepared veg, make your own mix from some of these sliced vegetables: broccoli, sugar snap peas, mushrooms, spring onions, carrots, beansprouts, or peppers.

Crab and noodle soup

50g/2oz thin rice noodles
100g/4oz Chinese-style stir-fry mixed
vegetables
2 tsp fish sauce
2 tsp sweet chilli sauce
600ml/1 pint vegetable stock
170g can white crabmeat in brine
a handful of coriander leaves,
roughly chopped, to garnish

Takes 8 minutes • Serves 2

1 Put the noodles and vegetables into a bowl, then pour over boiling water. Leave to soak for 4 minutes until the noodles are tender and the vegetables are just softened.
2 Heat together the fish sauce, chilli sauce and stock in a pan. Drain the noodles and veg from their soaking water and divide between two serving bowls. Add the crabmeat and pour over the hot stock. Scatter with coriander to serve.

• Per serving 184 kcalories, protein 17g, carbohydrate 28g, fat 1g, saturated fat none, fibre 3g, sugar 5g, salt 2.66g

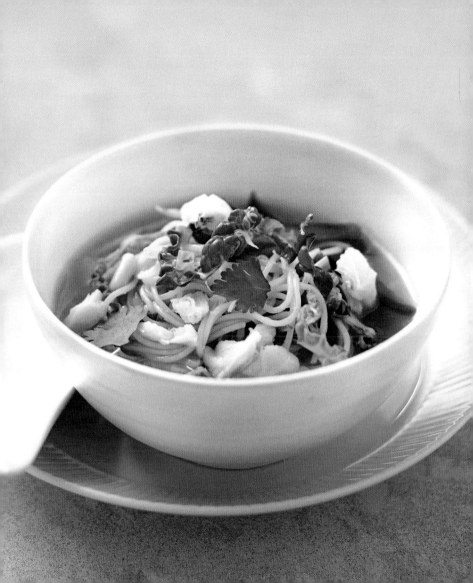

As well as supplying omega-3 fats, trout is an excellent
source of vitamin D, which is vital for strong bones.

Smoked trout and potato wedges

500g/1lb 2oz Maris Piper potatoes,
peeled and cubed
100g bag baby leaf spinach
zest and juice of 1 lemon
140g/5oz smoked trout fillet, flaked
1 tbsp capers
1 tbsp chopped dill
140g/5oz breadcrumbs,
from stale bread
1 tbsp sunflower oil
lemon wedges, tartare sauce and
green salad, to serve

Takes 40 minutes • Serves 4

1 Boil the potatoes in salted water for 15
minutes. Meanwhile, tip the spinach into a
large colander in the sink. Drain the potatoes
over the spinach so the cooking water wilts it,
then spoon the potatoes back into the pan.
Mash, stirring in the lemon zest and juice and
some seasoning, then fold through the trout
flakes, squeezed-out spinach, capers and dill.
2 Tip half the breadcrumbs on to a large
plate, then tip the potato mixture on to another
plate and shape into a large disc. Flip the
potato cake on to the crumbs, pressing the
remaining crumbs on to the top.
3 Heat the grill and pour the oil into a large
frying pan. Carefully slide the potato cake into
the pan, then cook for 5 minutes. Now grill for
4–5 minutes until golden and the cake is hot
through. Serve with lemon wedges, tartare
sauce and a green salad.

• Per serving 294 kcalories, protein 15g, carbohydrate
49g, fat 6g, saturated fat 1g, fibre 3g, sugar 2g,
salt 1.74g

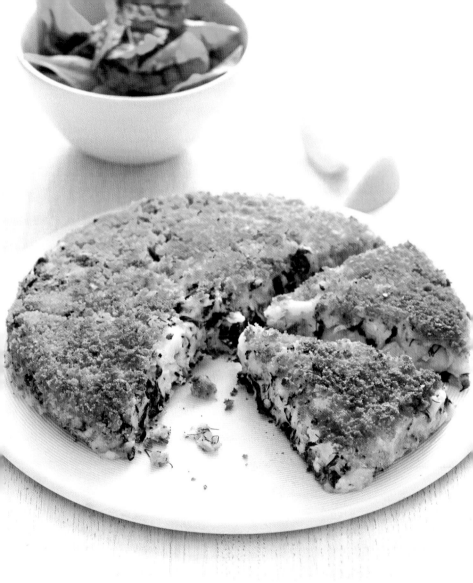

This recipe makes a great lunchbox salad to take to work. Soya beans are packed with nutrients; you'll find them in the vegetable section of the supermarket freezer cabinet.

Two bean, potato and tuna salad

300g/10oz new potatoes,
cut into chunks
175g/6oz green beans, trimmed
and halved
175g/6oz frozen soya beans
160g can tuna in water, drained well
a good handful of rocket or
watercress leaves, to garnish

FOR THE DRESSING
2 tsp harissa paste
1 tbsp red wine vinegar
2 tbsp olive oil

Takes 25 minutes • Serves 4

1 Put the potatoes in a pan of boiling water and cook for 6–8 minutes until almost tender. Add both types of beans, then boil for a further 5 minutes until everything is cooked.
2 Meanwhile, make the dressing. Whisk together the harissa and vinegar in a small bowl with a little seasoning. Whisk in the oil until the dressing is thickened. Drain the potatoes and beans well, toss with half of the dressing and leave to cool.
3 Flake the tuna, then fold into the potatoes and beans. Add the remaining dressing, then gently toss. Divide among four bowls and serve each portion with a handful of rocket or watercress leaves on top. Serve warm or cold.

• Per serving 211 kcalories, protein 15g, carbohydrate 19g, fat 9g, saturated fat 1g, fibre 4g, sugar 2g, salt 0.14g

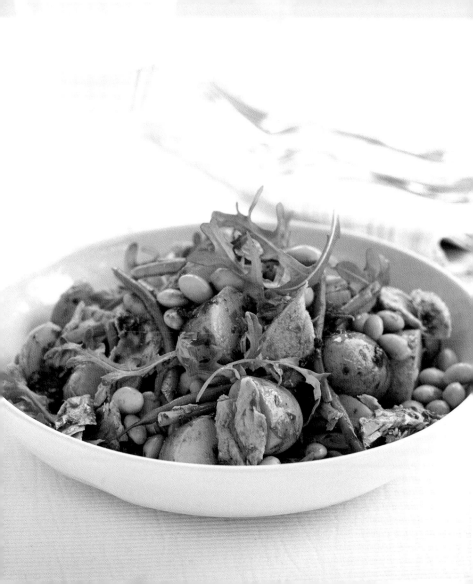

A good way to use up leftover pasta and make the most of spring's fresh new vegetables, like asparagus and broad beans. Ready in 10 minutes, this soup will become a favourite quick lunch.

Springtime minestrone

200g/8oz mixed green vegetables (asparagus, broad beans and spring onions)
700ml/1¼ pint hot vegetable stock
140g/5oz cooked pasta (spaghetti works well, chopped into small pieces)
215g can butter beans, drained and rinsed
3 tbsp green pesto

Takes 10 minutes • Serves 4

1 Put the green vegetables in a medium-sized pan, then pour over the stock. Bring to the boil, then reduce the heat and simmer until the vegetables are cooked through, about 3 minutes.

2 Stir in the cooked pasta, butter beans and 1 tablespoon of the pesto. Warm through, then ladle into bowls and top each with another drizzle of pesto.

• Per serving 125 kcalories, protein 8g, carbohydrate 16g, fat 4g, saturated fat 1g, fibre 4g, sugar 3g, salt 0.7g

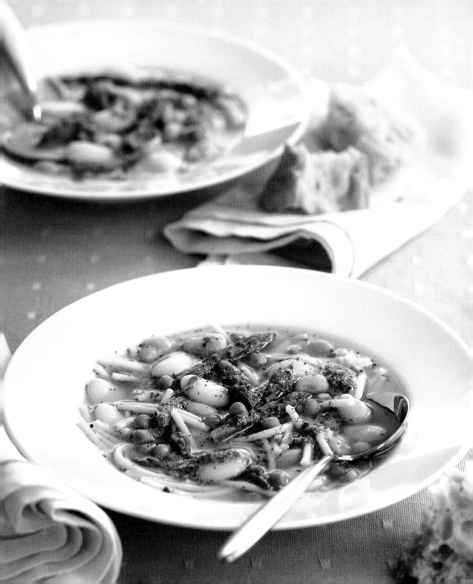

Just toss this together and serve on its own or with steamed rice or boiled noodles, if you like. As well as prawns you could flake leftover roast chicken through the salad.

Asian prawn & pineapple salad

1 small pineapple or 350g/12oz pineapple chunks
140g/5oz beansprouts
250g/9oz cooked peeled king prawns
½ cucumber, peeled, seeded and sliced on the angle
200g/8oz cherry tomatoes, halved
a handful of mint leaves, roughly chopped
50g/2oz unsalted cashew nuts, toasted

FOR THE DRESSING
½ red chilli, seeded and sliced
1 garlic clove
1 tsp golden caster sugar
juice of 2 limes
1½ tsp fish sauce

Takes 20 minutes • Serves 4

1 Mash the chilli, garlic and sugar to a paste using a pestle and mortar or small processor. Stir in the lime juice and fish sauce, then set the dressing aside.

2 Peel, quarter, core and slice the pineapple at an angle. Toss with beansprouts, prawns, cucumber and tomatoes and some of the dressing. Pile into bowls and scatter with mint and cashews. Drizzle with the rest of the dressing and serve.

• Per serving 202 kcalories, protein 19g, carbohydrate 17g, fat 7g, saturated fat 1g, fibre 3g, sugar 14g, salt 1.5g

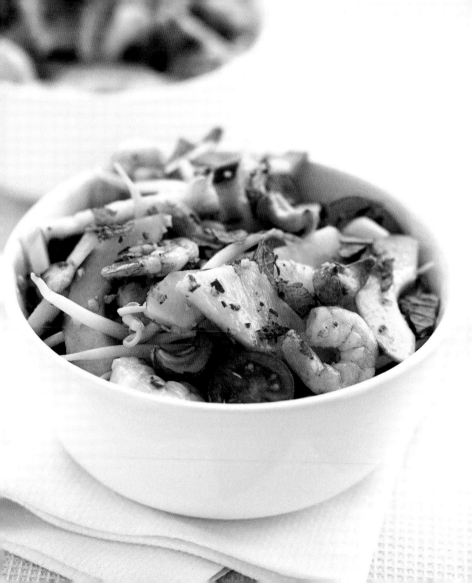

Fresh sage and apple are a classic flavour combination for pork, and choosing a quick-cook lean cut means this impressive-looking dish is ready in just 20 minutes. Serve with your favourite green veg.

Grilled pork with apple and sage

1 lemon
4 pieces pork tenderloin, about 140g/5oz each
2 tbsp roughly chopped sage leaves
3 eating apples, peeled, cored and chopped
1 rounded tbsp light muscovado sugar
green veg, to serve

Takes 20 minutes • Serves 4

1 Preheat the grill to high. Grate the zest from half the lemon and squeeze the juice from both halves. Split the pork fillets down the centre, cutting almost all the way through, and open each one out like a book. Lift on to a baking sheet and season with salt, pepper and the lemon zest. Sprinkle with 1 tablespoon of the sage. Grill for 8–10 minutes, turning once, until cooked through.
2 Meanwhile, pour the lemon juice into a small pan. Add the apples to the pan with the remaining sage, the sugar and salt and pepper to taste. Bring to the boil, stirring, then simmer until soft, about 6 minutes. Serve the pork and apples with a green veg of your choice.

• Per serving 269 kcalories, protein 31g, carbohydrate 16g, fat 9g, saturated fat 3g, fibre 1g, sugar 16g, salt 0.2g

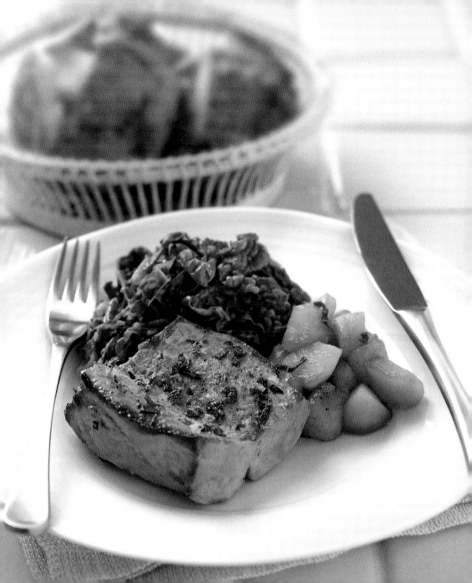

You can make this tasty low-fat salad all year round – just use a 198g can of drained sweetcorn instead of the fresh corn cobs.

Smoky chicken with warm corn and potato salad

500g bag new potatoes
2 large corn cobs
½ red onion, thinly sliced
juice of 1 lime
2 tbsp olive oil
2 garlic cloves, crushed
½–1 tsp sweet smoked paprika
4 skinless chicken breasts, each halved horizontally through the middle to make 2 thin escalopes
1 small bunch coriander, leaves roughly chopped
lime wedges, to serve

Takes 20 minutes • Serves 4

1 Bring to the boil a pan of water big enough to hold all the potatoes and corn. Cook the potatoes for 12 minutes, add the corn after 6 minutes, and boil until both are tender. Drain well.

2 Meanwhile, mix the onion with the lime juice and half the oil in a large salad bowl. Mix the remaining oil with the garlic, paprika and some seasoning in a shallow bowl, then toss in the chicken until thoroughly coated.

3 Heat a griddle pan and cook the chicken for 3 minutes on each side until cooked through. Tip the potatoes into the bowl with the onions. Stand a corn cob on one end on a chopping board, then slice down the length, cutting off the kernels in strips. Mix into the potato salad with the coriander and seasoning, then serve with the griddled chicken and lime wedges.

• Per serving 343 kcalories, protein 38g, carbohydrate 31g, fat 8g, saturated fat 1g, fibre 2g, sugar 4g, salt 0.25g

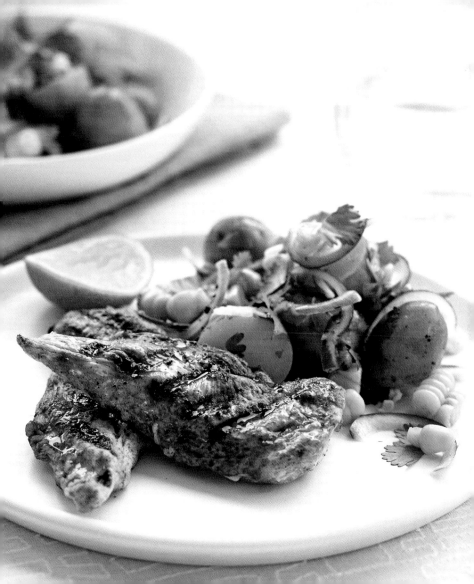

Just five simple ingredients, easy to cook and on the table in 10 minutes – what more could you want for a delicious home-from-work supper?

Thai beef stir-fry

2 tbsp vegetable oil
400g/14oz beef strips or steak cut into thin strips
1 red chilli, seeded and finely sliced
2 tbsp oyster sauce
a handful of basil leaves, to garnish
plain rice, to serve

Takes 10 minutes • Serves 4

1 Heat a wok or a large frying pan until smoking hot. Pour in the oil and swirl around the pan, then tip in the beef strips and chilli. Cook, stirring all the time, until the meat is lightly browned, about 3 minutes, then pour over the oyster sauce.
2 Cook until heated through and the sauce coats the meat. Garnish with the basil leaves and serve with plain rice.

• Per serving 178 kcalories, protein 22g, carbohydrate 1g, fat 10g, saturated fat 2g, fibre none, sugar 1g, salt 0.55g

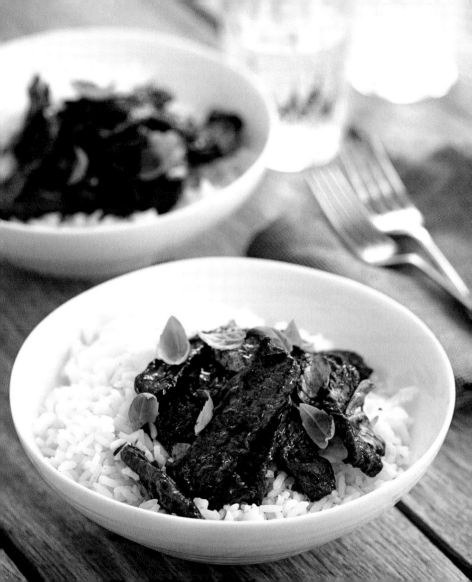

The crunchy cucumber and fennel salad mixed with Greek yogurt makes a perfect accompaniment to the juicy grilled kebabs.

Lamb kebabs with fennel and cucumber slaw

400g can green lentils,
drained and rinsed
250g pack lean minced lamb
1 tsp ground coriander
1 cucumber, chopped
1 fennel bulb, shredded
200g pot reduced-fat Greek yogurt
1 small garlic clove, crushed
(optional)
1 mild red chilli, seeded
and chopped

Takes 20 minutes • Serves 4

1 Preheat the grill to high. Put the lentils into the bowl of a food processor, then whiz to a rough paste. Tip into a bowl, add the mince, coriander and plenty of seasoning, then mix well. Roll into sixteen balls, divide them between four skewers and thread them on, then grill for 10 minutes, turning halfway through, until golden and juicy in the middle.
2 Meanwhile, mix the cucumber and fennel with the yogurt, garlic (if using), chilli and salt and pepper to taste. Serve with the kebabs.

• Per serving 202 kcalories, protein 21g, carbohydrate 12g, fat 8g, saturated fat 4g, fibre 3g, sugar 4g, salt 1.02g

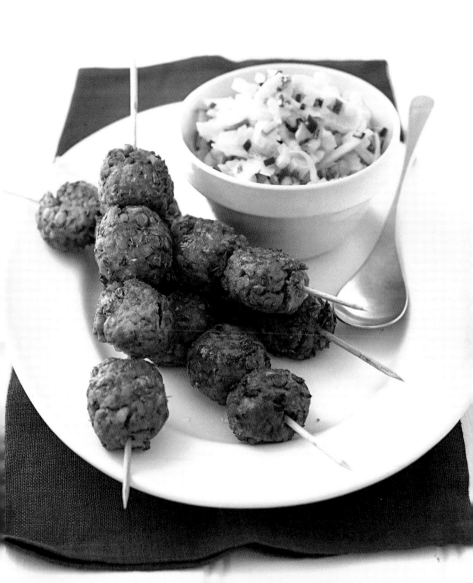

Adding corn to these healthy fish burgers makes them a hit with children and adults alike. Top with a good dollop of spicy tomato salsa for a scrummy supper.

Tuna sweetcorn burgers

85g/3oz white bread, torn into pieces
198g can sweetcorn, drained
2 × 185g cans tuna in water, drained well
25g/1oz grated Cheddar
3 spring onions, finely chopped
1 egg, beaten
2 tbsp vegetable oil
wholemeal buns, lettuce and salsa, to serve

Takes 15 minutes • Serves 4

1 Whiz the bread to crumbs in a food processor, tip into a bowl, then whiz half the sweetcorn until finely chopped. Add the chopped corn, remaining whole corn, tuna, cheese, spring onions and some seasoning to the bowl and mix well. Add the egg, bit by bit (you may not need it all), until the mixture is sticky enough to be shaped into four even-sized burgers.
2 Heat the oil in a non-stick pan, then cook the burgers for 5 minutes on each side until golden and hot through the middle.
3 Stuff into wholemeal buns with your favourite lettuce and some salsa to serve.

• Per serving 262 kcalories, protein 22g, carbohydrate 21g, fat 11g, saturated fat 3g, fibre 1g, sugar 5g, salt 0.87g

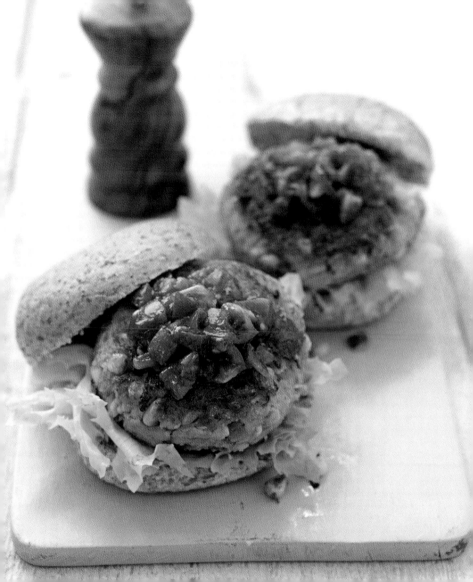

Full of delicious sweetness, this healthy dish is a good source of vitamin C and iron. You can use vegetable stock instead of water for the couscous.

Sticky chicken with mango couscous

1 large mango
4 spring onions, sliced
1 heaped tsp ground cumin
3 tbsp white wine vinegar
250g/9oz couscous
3 tbsp thick-cut marmalade
4 tsp grainy mustard
4 chicken breasts, each sliced
into 3–4 strips

Takes 20 minutes • Serves 4

1 Preheat the grill to high. Peel and dice the mango, toss with most of the spring onions, and the cumin and vinegar, then set aside. Put the couscous in a large heatproof bowl, pour over 400ml/14fl oz boiling water, then cover with cling film and set aside.
2 Mix together the marmalade and mustard. Lay the chicken strips in a roasting tin, then brush over half of the marmalade glaze. Grill for 4–5 minutes, then turn the chicken over and brush with the remaining glaze. Grill for a further 4–5 minutes until the chicken is cooked through, and the glaze is bubbling.
3 The couscous should now be ready. Stir in the mango mixture and serve with the hot chicken strips and the remaining spring onions sprinkled over.

• Per serving 369 kcalories, protein 35g, carbohydrate 53g, fat 3g, saturated fat 1g, fibre 3g, sugar 21g, salt 0.43g

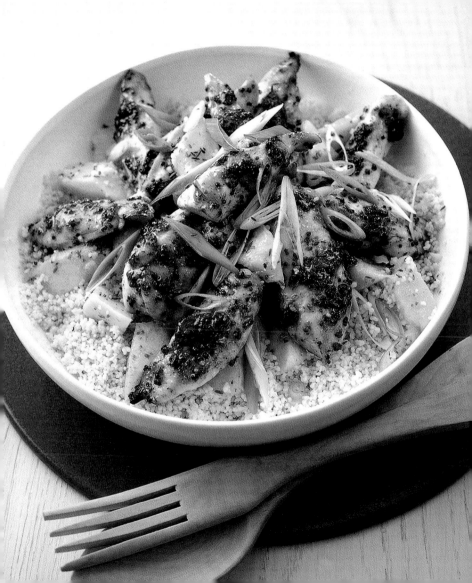

The subtle hint of mustard complements the pork in this dish.
A good supper idea for family or friends and great served
with mash and vegetables.

Mustardy pork and apples

4 pork steaks, about 140g/5oz each,
trimmed of excess fat
1 tbsp oil
2 eating apples, cored and cut into
eight (red-skinned look good)
1 onion, halved and sliced
a small handful of sage leaves, torn,
or 2 tsp dried
100ml/3½fl oz chicken stock
(from a cube is fine)
2 tsp wholegrain or Dijon mustard
mash and green veg, to serve

Takes 25 minutes • Serves 4

1 Rub the pork steaks with a little oil and season with pepper and salt to taste. Heat a large frying pan and fry the steaks for 2 minutes on both sides until golden. Transfer to a plate.
2 Adding a little more oil to the pan, fry the apples, onion and sage for 5 minutes or until the apples have softened. Pour in the stock and spoon in the mustard, then return the pork to the pan and simmer for 10 minutes until the sauce has reduced by about a third and the pork is cooked through. Serve with mash and some green veg.

• Per serving 248 kcalories, protein 35g, carbohydrate 9g, fat 8g, saturated fat 2g, fibre 2g, sugar 8g, salt 0.42g

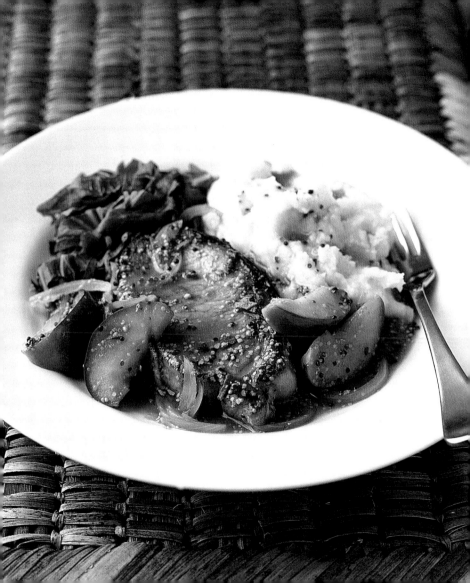

For extra crunch and colour, add a handful of walnut pieces and cranberries to the mince in this quick-cook, new-style meatloaf.

Turkey, thyme and leek meatloaf

1 tbsp sunflower oil
4 large leeks, sliced
500g pack minced turkey
2 thyme sprigs, leaves stripped
85g/3oz fresh breadcrumbs
1 egg, beaten
2 rashers lean back bacon, fat trimmed, chopped
boiled potatoes and carrots, to serve

Takes 30 minutes • Serves 4

1 Preheat the oven to 220°C/200°C fan/gas 7. Heat the oil in a frying pan, then soften the leeks for 5 minutes. Line the base of a 28x18cm baking tin with greaseproof paper.
2 Mix the mince, thyme, two-thirds of the breadcrumbs, the leeks and egg together with a little seasoning, then tip into the tin. Press the mixture firmly into the tin, then ruffle the surface with a fork. Mix the remaining breadcrumbs and the bacon together, and scatter over the top. Cook for 15 minutes, then finish under the grill until golden and crisp on top. Serve with boiled potatoes and carrots.

• Per serving 302 kcalories, protein 37g, carbohydrate 20g, fat 8g, saturated fat 2g, fibre 3g, sugar 3g, salt 1.20g

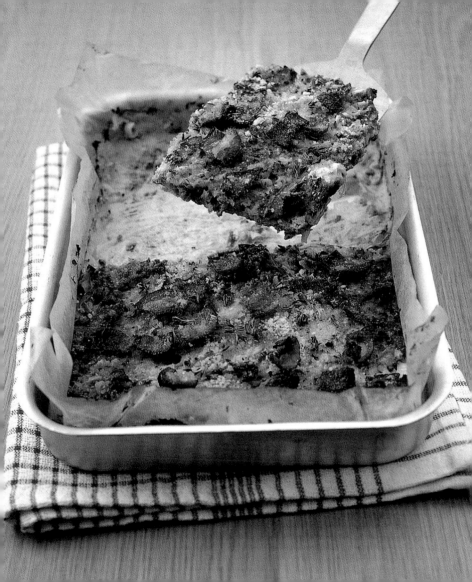

This fish pilaf is packed with goodness and makes a tasty and quick midweek supper.

Zesty lentil and haddock pilaf

250g/9oz easy-cook basmati rice
3 red onions, finely sliced
2 tbsp olive oil
140g/5oz smoked haddock fillet
140g/5oz haddock fillet
250g pack ready-cooked Puy lentils
zest of 1 lemon (then cut the lemon into wedges, to serve)
1 large bunch flatleaf parsley, leaves roughly chopped
25g/1oz toasted flaked almonds, to garnish

Takes 20 minutes • Serves 4

1 Cook the rice in boiling water until just tender, then drain.
2 Meanwhile, fry the onions in the oil in a large non-stick frying pan over a medium heat for 10–12 minutes until golden.
3 Bring some water to the boil in a shallow pan. Add the haddock fillets, poach for 4 minutes until the fish is just cooked, then drain and break into large flakes.
4 Spoon half the onions on to a plate, then set aside. Stir the drained rice and lentils into the onion pan, then fold through the fish, lemon zest and parsley to heat through. Serve topped with the reserved onions and the almonds, with the lemon wedges on the side for squeezing over.

• Per serving 468 kcalories, protein 27g, carbohydrate 70g, fat 11g, saturated fat 1g, fibre 7g, sugar 6g, salt 1.39g

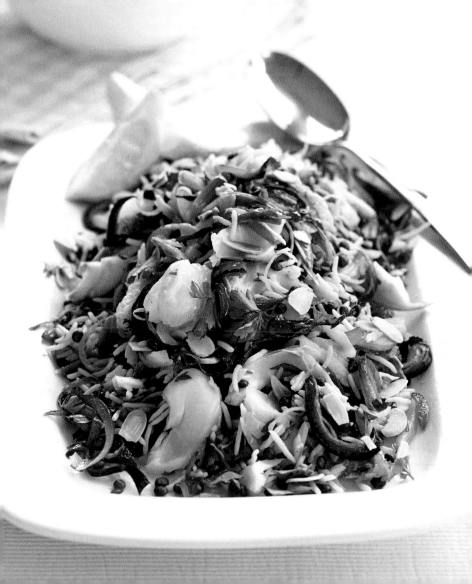

Rump steak is a good choice for this dish as it's not too expensive and has plenty of flavour. Trim off any excess fat after grilling. Some steamed rice flavoured with rice vinegar is a good accompaniment.

Beef strips with crunchy Thai salad

2 thick-cut lean steaks, about
600g/1lb 5oz in total
4 tbsp fresh lime juice
1 tbsp Thai fish sauce
1 tbsp light muscovado sugar
1 red chilli, seeded and
finely chopped
200g bag crunchy salad mix
50g/2oz carrot, grated
a handful of beansprouts

Takes 10 minutes • Serves 4

1 Heat the grill to high. Lightly season the steaks, then grill on each side for 2–3 minutes for medium-rare, or longer if you prefer your meat more well done.
2 Mix the lime juice, fish sauce, sugar and chilli together in a jug.
3 Tip the salad, carrot and beansprouts into a bowl, then add the dressing, tossing everything together. Divide among four plates.
4 Thinly slice the beef and add to the salad.

• Per serving 242 kcalories, protein 33g, carbohydrate 6g, fat 10g, saturated fat 4g, fibre 1g, sugar 6g, salt 0.92g

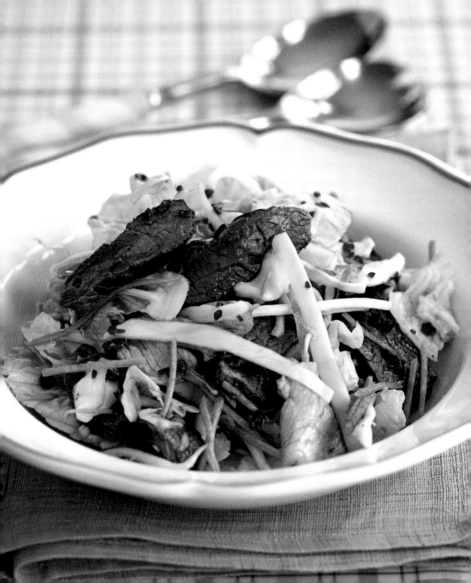

Root vegetables make a healthy alternative to potato. Celeriac is rich in vitamin C and carrots in beta-carotene, which we convert to vitamin A.

Mustard chicken with celeriac and carrot mash

1 large celeriac, about 1kg/2lb 4oz, peeled
500g/1lb 2oz carrots
500g/1lb 2oz skinless chicken breasts
1 tbsp plain flour, seasoned with salt and pepper
1 tbsp sunflower oil
2 tbsp wholegrain mustard
300ml/½ pint vegetable or chicken stock
steamed green beans, to serve

Takes 20 minutes • Serves 4

1 Slice the celeriac and carrots in a food processor, then put in a pan and pour over boiling water to cover. Add a little salt, then cover and boil for 10–12 minutes until tender.
2 Meanwhile, cut the chicken into strips and toss in the seasoned flour. Heat the oil in a large frying pan, add the chicken and fry quickly on all sides until lightly browned. Stir in the mustard and stock, then bring to the boil. Simmer uncovered, stirring occasionally, for 5–6 minutes until the chicken is cooked and the sauce thickened.
3 Drain the veg and whiz to a rough mash. Divide among four plates with the chicken and sauce. Serve with steamed green beans.

• Per serving 248 kcalories, protein 34g, carbohydrate 16g, fat 6g, saturated fat 1g, fibre 9g, sugar 12g, salt 1.01g

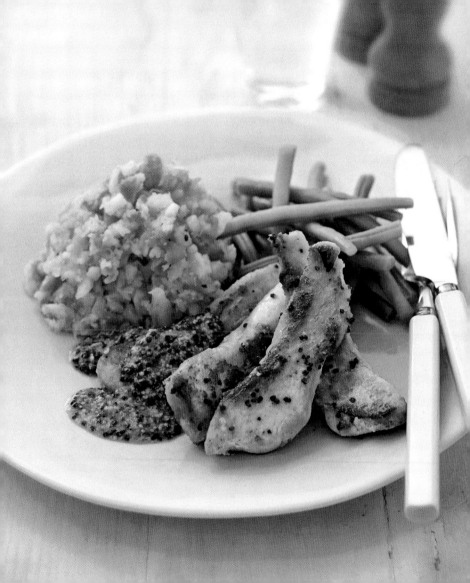

For a change, try swapping the couscous for bulghar wheat. It's just as quick to prepare and has a lovely nutty flavour that goes really well with citrusy dressings.

Smoky prawns with green couscous

200g/8oz large raw peeled prawns
zest and juice of 2 lemons, plus extra
wedges to serve
2 garlic cloves, crushed
2 tsp paprika
2 tbsp olive oil
175g/6oz couscous
4 courgettes, sliced on the diagonal
large bunch coriander, leaves only,
chopped

Takes 25 minutes • Serves 4

1 Tip the prawns into a small bowl. Add all the lemon zest, plus the juice from 1 lemon, the garlic, paprika and 1 tablespoon of oil. Mix, then set aside. Put the couscous into a large bowl, pour over 250ml/9fl oz boiling water, cover and set aside for 10 minutes.
2 Heat a non-stick frying pan, then add 1 tablespoon of the prawn marinade, the courgettes and a splash of water. Stir-fry for 4–5 minutes until the courgettes are golden, then tip on to a plate and set aside. Add the prawns to the pan with their marinade, then fry for 1 minute until just pink.
3 Fluff up the couscous with a fork, then mix in the courgettes, coriander, remaining oil and lemon juice and some seasoning. Lastly, scrape in the prawns with all the pan juices and toss briefly before serving with extra lemon wedges for squeezing.

• Per serving 219 kcalories, protein 14g, carbohydrate 26g, fat 7g, saturated fat 1g, fibre 1g, sugar 3g, salt 0.26g

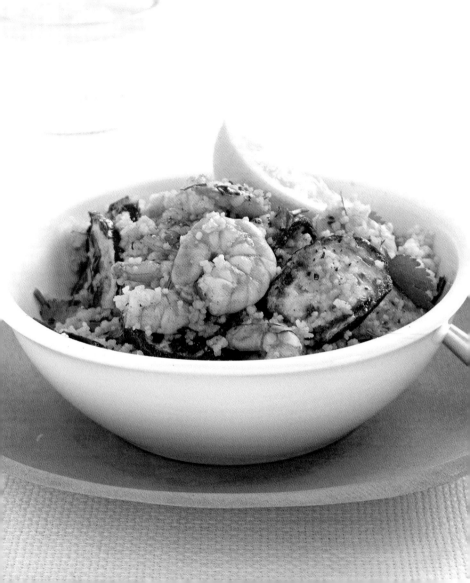

Make the 16 koftas and then freeze half of them, uncooked, for supper or lunch on another day. Children love these meatballs served with wraps and a crunchy salad.

Lemon and cumin koftas

1kg/2lb 4oz lean minced lamb
zest and juice of 2 lemons
small bunch mint, leaves only,
roughly chopped (save a little for
the salad)
4 tsp ground cumin
1 garlic clove, crushed

FOR THE CABBAGE SALAD
½ small red cabbage
1 red onion
1 tsp sugar
wraps or flatbreads and ready-made
raita or tzatziki, to serve

Takes 30 minutes • Makes 16

1 Preheat the grill to medium. Put the mince in a large bowl and add the lemon zest, half of the juice, most of the mint, cumin, garlic and seasoning to taste. Use your hands to mix well, then shape into 16 evenly sized balls, and set aside on a plate. (Freeze half at this stage.)
2 Grill the koftas for 12–15 minutes on a grill rack, turning once, until well browned.
3 Meanwhile, make the salad: shred the cabbage and finely slice the onion, then toss with the remaining lemon juice, sugar, reserved mint and seasoning to taste.
4 Serve two koftas per person, in wraps or flatbreads, with the salad and some raita or tzatziki.

• Per serving 217 kcalories, protein 27g, carbohydrate 4g, fat 11g, saturated fat 5g, fibre 1g, sugar 3g, salt 0.24g

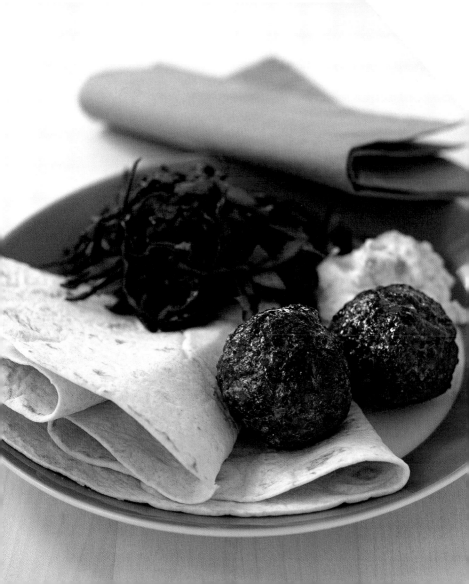

our veg count by adding a handful of any of the following
af: broad beans, peas, grated courgette, shredded leeks,
sweetcorn or some chopped red pepper.

Coriander cod with carrot pilaf

2 tbsp olive oil
4 skinless cod fillets, about
175g/6oz each
2 tbsp chopped coriander
zest and juice of 1 lemon
1 onion, chopped
2 tsp cumin seeds
2 large carrots, grated
200g/8oz basmati rice
600ml/1 pint vegetable stock

Takes 25 minutes • Serves 4

1 Preheat the grill to high, then line the grill pan with a double thickness of foil and curl up the edges to catch the juices. Brush lightly with a little of the oil and put the cod on top. Sprinkle over the coriander, lemon zest and juice, and drizzle with a little more of the oil. Season with salt and pepper, then grill for 10–12 minutes until the fish flakes easily.
2 Meanwhile, heat the remaining oil in a pan. Add the onion and cumin seeds, and fry for a few minutes. Add the carrots and stir well, then stir in the rice until glistening. Add the stock and bring to the boil. Cover and cook gently for about 10 minutes until the rice is tender and the stock absorbed. Spoon the rice on to four warm plates, top with the cod and pour over the pan juices.

• Per serving 305 kcalories, protein 14g, carbohydrate 50g, fat 7g, saturated fat 1g, fibre 3g, sugar 8g, salt 0.31g

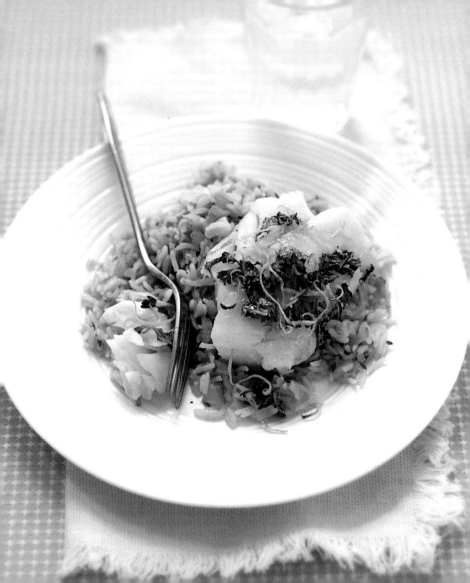

The pepperiness of watercress works extremely well with Asian flavours, and this main-dish salad is a good example. If you like cucumber, add some chunks to give extra low-fat crunchiness.

Asian beef and watercress salad

500g/1lb 2oz lean stir-fry beef, cubed
3 tsp fish sauce
juice of 2 limes
small knob of ginger, peeled and finely chopped
1 garlic clove, crushed
1 small red chilli, seeded and finely chopped
2 tbsp soft brown sugar
2 bunches watercress
1 mango, peeled and cut into medium chunks
1 small red onion, thinly sliced into half moons
1 tsp vegetable oil

Takes 30 minutes • Serves 4

1 Season the beef with some pepper and 1 teaspoon of the fish sauce and set aside.
2 In a small bowl, mix together the lime juice, ginger, garlic, chilli, brown sugar and remaining fish sauce. Taste for extra fish sauce or sugar – it should be sweet, salty and sour without any one being dominant.
3 Place a handful of watercress on each serving plate, then divide the mango chunks and red onion among them.
4 Just before serving, set a wok over a high heat and tip in the oil. Sear the meat, turning often until browned all over. Divide among the plates of salad and pour the dressing over. Serve while warm.

• Per serving 255 kcalories, protein 30g, carbohydrate 20g, fat 6g, saturated fat 2g, fibre 3g, sugar 19g, salt 0.98g

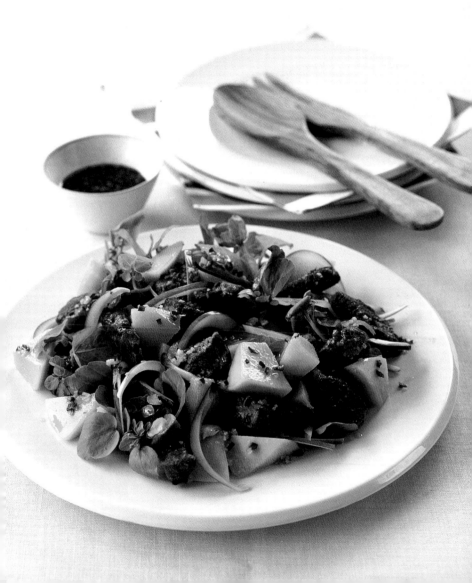

To make sure the avocado you buy is ripe for this fresh-tasting salad, look for one with dark green skin and gently squeeze to check it is soft.

Chicken with warm orange and avocado salsa

2 tsp olive oil

4 skinless chicken breasts, cut in half on the diagonal

zest and juice of 1 lime

1 avocado

2 oranges

1 red chilli, seeded and diced (optional)

3 spring onions, finely sliced

1 tbsp chopped coriander or basil

Takes 20 minutes • Serves 4

1 Heat the oil in a non-stick frying pan, season the chicken and fry for 10 minutes, turning once. Add the lime juice for the final minute of cooking.

2 Meanwhile, halve the avocado and remove the stone. Peel away the skin and use a small knife to cut the flesh into small chunks. Tip into a bowl. Cut away the skin and pith of the oranges, cut out the segments, then add to the avocado with the remaining ingredients, not forgetting the lime zest. Toss gently, then serve alongside the chicken.

• Per serving 240 kcalories, protein 35g, carbohydrate 8g, fat 8g, saturated fat 1g, fibre 3g, sugar 7g, salt 0.23g

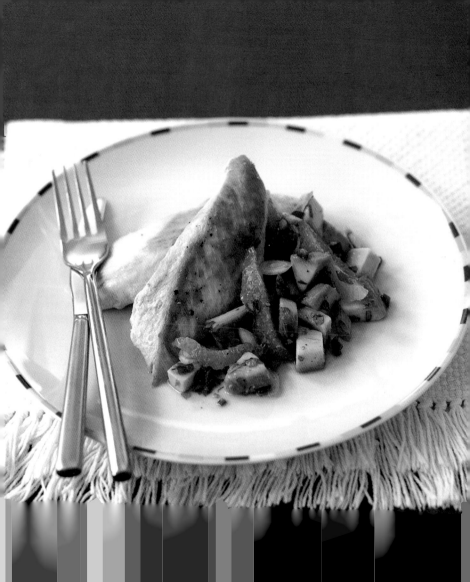

Who needs a take-away when this home-cooked version of a popular favourite is so easy to make?

Egg-fried rice with prawns and peas

250g/9oz basmati rice
2 tbsp vegetable oil
2 garlic cloves, finely chopped
1 red chilli, seeded and shredded
2 eggs, beaten
200g/8oz frozen peas
1 bunch spring onions, finely sliced
285g pack cooked peeled
small prawns
1 tbsp soy sauce, plus extra
to serve (optional)

Takes 25 minutes • Serves 4

1 Put the rice in a pan with 600ml/1 pint water. Bring to the boil, cover, then simmer for 10 minutes or until almost all the water has gone. Leave off the heat, covered, for 5 minutes more.
2 Heat the oil in a wok or large frying pan. Add the garlic and chilli, then cook for just 10 seconds – making sure not to let it burn. Throw in the cooked rice, stir-fry for 1 minute, then push to the side of the pan. Pour the eggs into the empty side of the pan, then scramble them, stirring.
3 Once just set, stir the peas and spring onions into the rice and egg, then cook for 2 minutes until the peas are tender. Add the prawns and soy sauce, heat through, then serve with extra soy sauce on the side, if you like.

• Per serving 416 kcalories, protein 28g, carbohydrate 56g, fat 10g, saturated fat 2g, fibre 3g, sugar 2g, salt 2.06g

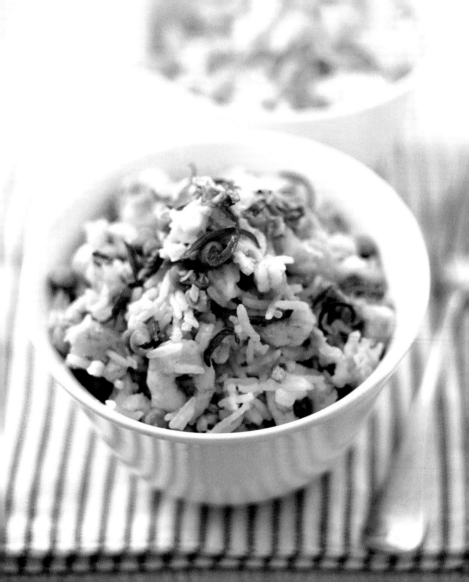

The citrus zest and juice adds a refreshing zing to this casserole.
Serve with a bowl of fluffy mash sprinkled with chopped parsley.

Sticky lemon pork

3 tbsp plain flour
1 tbsp paprika
800g/1lb 12oz leg or shoulder of
pork, diced into large chunks
2 tbsp olive oil
2 rosemary sprigs, leaves stripped
4 garlic cloves, chopped
3 bay leaves
300ml/½ pint white wine
peeled zest and juice of 1 lemon

Takes 1 hour 40 minutes • Serves 4

1 Tip the flour, paprika, salt and pepper into a food bag and toss in the pork until coated. Heat the oil in a flameproof casserole and fry the pork until brown on all sides. Add the rosemary, garlic and bay leaves, then fry for 1 minute more. Pour in the wine and bring to the boil, scraping the bottom of the casserole to remove any bits. Lower to a simmer and throw in the lemon zest.

2 Cover the casserole, place on the lowest heat and simmer for 1 hour until the pork is tender. Add a splash of water if the sauce becomes too thick. Just before serving, stir in the lemon juice and check the seasoning.

• Per serving 356 kcalories, protein 46g, carbohydrate 14g, fat 11g, saturated fat 3g, fibre 1g, sugar 4g, salt 0.34g

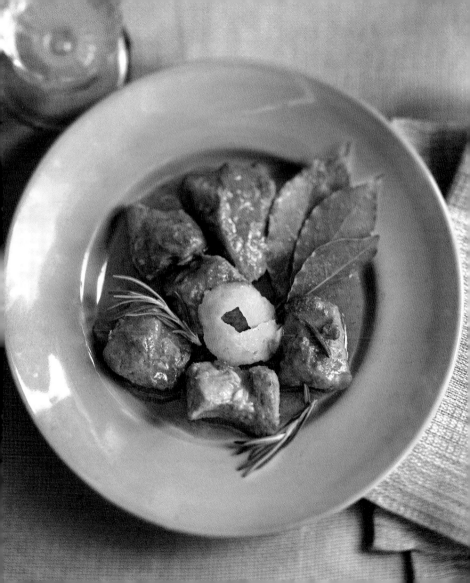

This speedy biryani is so simple to make. The spinach is an unusual addition that is stirred in for the last 5 minutes, but it adds a wonderful flavour and texture.

Quick lamb biryani

1 tbsp balti curry paste
500g/1lb 2oz lean lamb leg steak or neck fillet, cubed
200g/8oz basmati rice, rinsed in cold water
400ml/14fl oz lamb or chicken stock
250g bag spinach leaves

Takes 25 minutes • Serves 4

1 Heat a large pan and fry the curry paste until fragrant. Add the lamb and brown it on all sides. Pour in the rice and stock, then stir well. Bring to the boil, cover with a lid, then cook for 15 minutes on a medium heat until the rice is tender.

2 Stir through the spinach, put the lid back on the pan and leave to steam, undisturbed, for 5 minutes before serving.

• Per serving 387 kcalories, protein 32g, carbohydrate 41g, fat 12g, saturated fat 5g, fibre 1g, sugar 1g, salt 1.05g

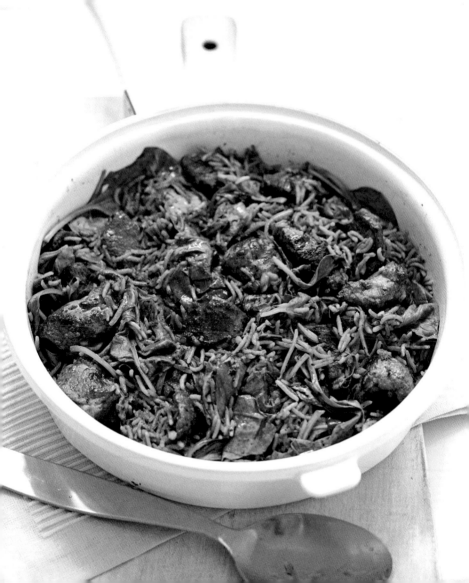

Coating the chicken in cornflour before frying helps it not only to crisp it up, but also to thicken the sauce.

Sticky lemon chicken

1 tbsp clear honey
juice of 1 lemon
250ml/9fl oz chicken stock
1 tbsp soy sauce
4 chicken breasts, cut into chunks
1 tbsp cornflour
1 tsp vegetable oil
2 carrots, finely sliced
1 red pepper, seeded and
cut into chunks
140g/5oz sugar snap peas
noodles, to serve

Takes 30 minutes • Serves 4

1 In a jug, mix together the honey, lemon, stock and soy sauce, then set aside. Toss the chicken with the cornflour so it is completely coated. Heat the oil in a non-stick frying pan, then fry the chicken until it changes colour and starts to become crisp around the edges.
2 Add the carrots and red pepper, then fry for 1 minute more. Pour the stock mixture into the pan, bring to a simmer, then add the sugar snap peas and bubble everything together for 5 minutes until the chicken is cooked and the vegetables are tender. Serve with noodles.

• Per serving 236 kcalories, protein 38g, carbohydrate 15g, fat 3g, saturated fat 1g, fibre 2g, sugar 10g, salt 1.25g

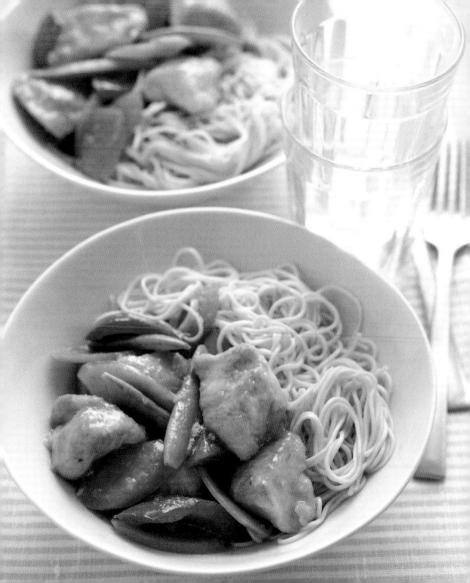

This easy risotto is baked in the oven rather than stirred on the hob while you add the stock bit by bit – the result tastes just as good.

Oven-baked red pepper risotto

1 tbsp oil
1 onion, chopped
300g/10oz risotto rice
100ml/3½fl oz white wine (optional, or use more stock)
400g can chopped tomatoes
200g/8oz frozen roasted peppers
500ml/18fl oz vegetable stock
a handful of flatleaf parsley, chopped
Parmesan, to garnish (optional)

Takes 35 minutes • Serves 4

1 Preheat the oven to 200°C/180°C fan/gas 6. Heat the oil in an ovenproof pan, then fry the onion for a few minutes until softened. Turn up the heat, tip in the rice, stir, then fry for 1 minute more.

2 Pour in the wine, if using, or more stock, stirring until absorbed, then tip in the tomatoes, peppers and 400ml/14fl oz of the stock. Cover and bake in the oven for 25 minutes until the rice is tender and creamy.

3 Stir in the remaining stock and the parsley, season and scatter with Parmesan shavings, if you like.

• Per serving 334 kcalories, protein 9g, carbohydrate 70g, fat 4g, saturated fat 1g, fibre 5g, sugar 9g, salt 1.36g

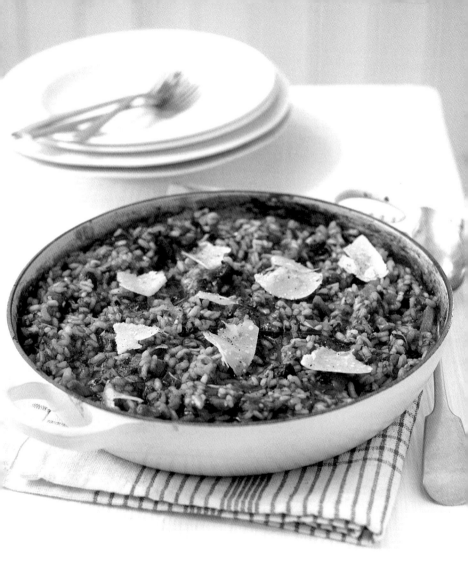

If you take the skin off chicken before cooking it dramatically reduces the saturated fat content. Removing the skin also shaves 10 minutes off the cooking time.

Chicken with wine and mushrooms

4 skinless chicken breasts
1 tbsp plain flour, seasoned
150ml/¼ pint chicken stock
(use ½ a cube)
1 tbsp mild olive or vegetable oil
250g pack chestnut mushrooms,
halved
a few thyme sprigs
150ml/¼ pint red wine
mash, to serve

Takes 20 minutes • Serves 4

1 Toss the chicken in the flour, then tap off the excess. Mix 1 teaspoon of the excess flour with a little stock and set aside. Heat the oil in a frying pan, then add the chicken, mushrooms and thyme. Cook over a medium–high heat for about 5 minutes, turning the chicken breasts once until golden all over.

2 Lift the chicken out, then set aside. Pour in the wine and the remaining stock, and boil for 5 minutes or until reduced by half. Add the flour-and-stock mix, stirring until the sauce thickens a little. Put the chicken back into the pan, along with any juices from the plate, then simmer for 5 minutes or until cooked through and the sauce is glossy. Serve the chicken with mash.

• Per serving 216 kcalories, protein 35g, carbohydrate 5g, fat 5g, saturated fat 1g, fibre 1g, sugar 2g, salt 0.99g

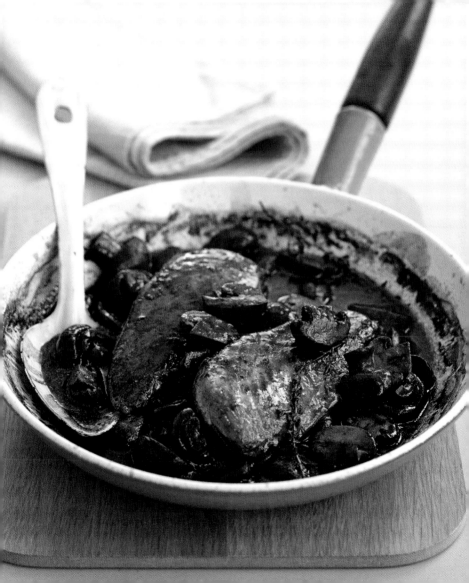

Ultra-thin minute steak is great for weeknight suppers
because it's quick to cook. It is also very lean, so
lower in fat than other cuts of beef.

Goulash in a dash

1 tbsp vegetable oil
300g/10oz stir-fry beef strips or
minute steak, cut into strips
100g/4oz chestnut mushrooms,
quartered
2 tsp paprika
500g/1lb 2oz potatoes, peeled and
cut into smallish chunks
600ml/1 pint hot beef stock (a cube
is fine)
500g jar tomato-based cooking
sauce
a handful of parsley leaves,
roughly chopped
natural yogurt, to garnish
crusty bread or rice, to serve

Takes 30 minutes • Serves 4

1 Heat half the oil in a large non-stick pan and fry the beef for 2 minutes, stirring once halfway through. Tip the meat on to a plate. Heat the remaining oil in the pan (there is no need to clean it) and fry the mushrooms for 2–3 minutes until they start to colour.
2 Sprinkle the paprika over the mushrooms, fry briefly, then tip in potatoes, stock and tomato sauce. Give it all a good stir, then cover and simmer for 20 minutes until the potatoes are tender. Return the beef to the pan along with any juices, and warm through. Stir in the parsley and a swirl of yogurt, then serve straight from the pan. Crusty bread or rice make a good accompaniment.

• Per serving 299 kcalories, protein 23g, carbohydrate 33g, fat 9g, saturated fat 2g, fibre 3g, sugar 5g, salt 1.59g

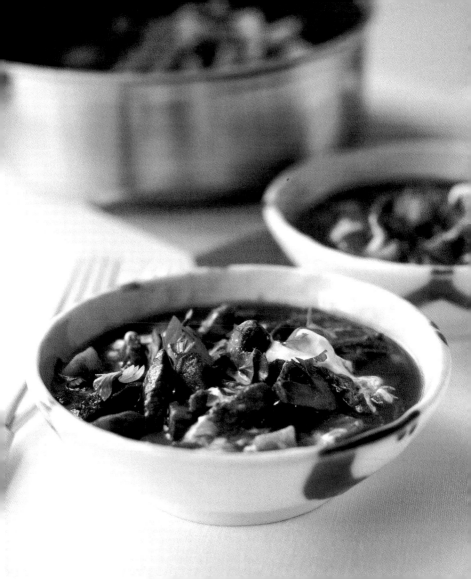

Fresh crab is one of summer's real treats and its delicate flavour means it needs only minimal cooking. This pasta dish is ready on the table in just 15 minutes.

Creamy crab and pea pasta

400g/14oz spaghetti
200g/8oz fresh or frozen peas
300g/10oz fresh crabmeat
5 tbsp reduced-fat crème fraîche
juice of ½ lemon
1 red chilli, seeded and chopped, plus extra to garnish
a handful of parsley leaves, chopped
zest of 1 lemon, to garnish

Takes 15 minutes • Serves 4

1 Boil a large pan of salted water. Tip in the pasta, then cook for about 7 minutes. Add the peas, then cook for 2–3 minutes more until both are cooked through.
2 Drain in a colander, reserving a little cooking water, then tip back into the pan with the crabmeat and crème fraîche. Stir it all together well with the lemon juice, most of the chilli and parsley and a little of the pasta cooking water if the mixture seems dry. Serve sprinkled with the remaining chilli and parsley and the lemon zest.

• Per serving 512 kcalories, protein 31g, carbohydrate 81g, fat 10g, saturated fat 3g, fibre 5g, sugar 5g, salt 0.83g

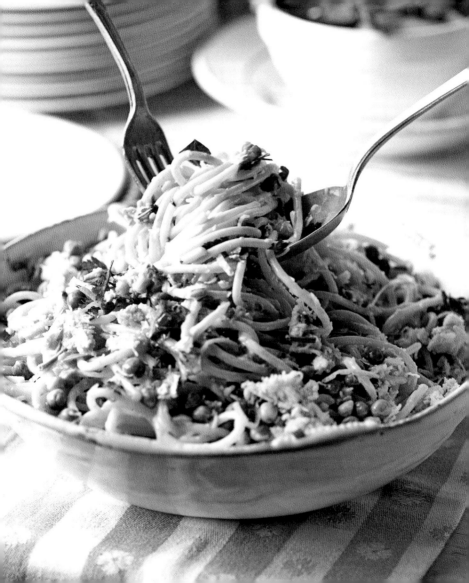

Beef stir-fry strips are handy, but you can also slice your own steaks instead. Put them in the freezer for 10 minutes then cut into slices.

Beef stir-fry with broccoli and oyster sauce

1–2 tbsp sunflower oil
200g/8oz beef stir-fry strips
200g pack Tenderstem broccoli
1 onion, sliced
2 garlic cloves, sliced
2 tbsp oyster sauce

Takes 15 minutes • Serves 2

1 Heat a wok until smoking, pour in the oil then add the beef. Stir-fry for 2 minutes, then tip the beef on to a plate. Add the broccoli with a splash of water then cook until it turns bright green.
2 Add the onion and stir-fry for 1 minute, then add the garlic and cook for 1 minute more. Pour in the oyster sauce and 125ml/4fl oz water. Bring to the boil and cook until reduced to a sticky sauce. Stir in the beef, along with any juices from the plate, then serve straight away.

• Per serving 256 kcalories, protein 30g, carbohydrate 10g, fat 12g, saturated fat 2g, fibre 4g, sugar 8g, salt 1.78g

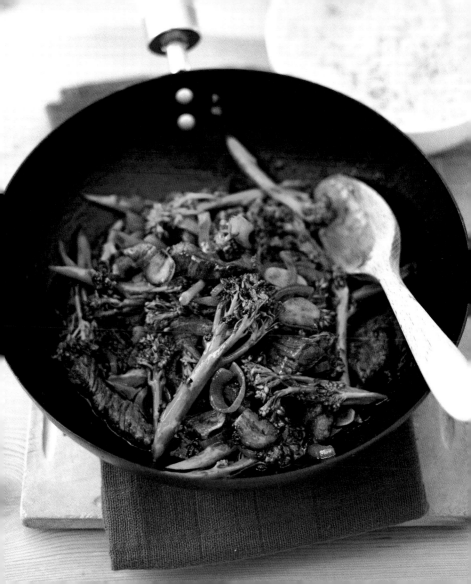

Use roasted or boiled beetroot for this dish; if buying it cooked, go for vac-packed, but make sure it's not pickled in vinegar. Serve with fried eggs for brunch.

Red flannel hash

800g/1lb 12oz boiled potatoes
3 tbsp sunflower oil
140g/5oz corned beef, shredded
3 cooked beetroots, peeled and diced
horseradish sauce, to serve

Takes 35 minutes • Serves 4

1 Break up the potatoes. Heat the oil in a heavy frying pan, then add the potatoes and corned beef, and cook, turning the potato chunks over with a fish slice every time they become crisp.

2 After about 10 minutes, when the potatoes are crisp all over, stir through the beetroots, then season. Turn down the heat, pat the potatoes into a cake, then leave to brown on the bottom. Invert on to a plate, then return to the pan until the other side is browned.

3 Serve straight from the pan, or turn out on to a board and cut into wedges. Serve with the horseradish sauce.

• Per serving 303 kcalories, protein 13g, carbohydrate 37g, fat 12g, saturated fat 3g, fibre 3g, sugar 4g, salt 1.17g

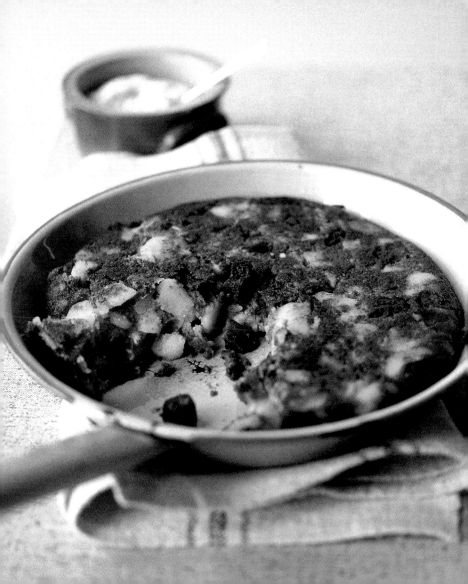

The combination of cinnamon, coriander and cumin with the lemon, chickpeas and chicken makes this a perfectly balanced meal. Serve with lots of crusty bread to mop up the sauce.

Lemon-spiced chicken with chickpeas

1 tbsp sunflower oil
1 onion, halved and thinly sliced
4 skinless chicken breasts,
cut into chunks
1 cinnamon stick, broken in half
1 tsp each ground coriander
and cumin
zest and juice of 1 lemon
400g can chickpeas, drained
and rinsed
200ml/7fl oz chicken stock
250g bag spinach leaves

Takes 20 minutes • Serves 4

1 Heat the oil in a large frying pan, then fry the onion gently for 5 minutes. Turn up the heat and add the chicken, frying for about 3 minutes until golden.
2 Stir in the spices and lemon zest, fry for 1 more minute, then tip in the chickpeas and stock. Put the lid on and simmer for 5 minutes. Season to taste, then tip in the spinach and re-cover. Leave to wilt for 2 minutes, then stir through. Squeeze over the lemon juice just before serving.

• Per serving 290 kcalories, protein 42g, carbohydrate 14g, fat 7g, saturated fat 1g, fibre 4g, sugar 3g, salt 1.03g

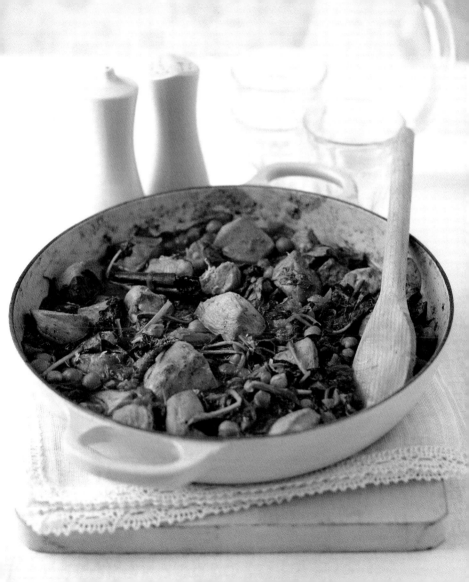

A clean, fresh-tasting dish that's packed with flavour
and includes three of your 5-a-day.

Prawn, pea and tomato curry

1 tbsp vegetable oil
2 onions, halved, each cut into 6 wedges
6 ripe tomatoes, each cut into 8 wedges
large knob of ginger, peeled and chopped
6 garlic cloves, roughly chopped
3 tbsp curry paste (we used tikka masala paste)
400g/14oz peeled raw king prawns
250g/9oz frozen peas
1 small bunch coriander, leaves chopped, to garnish
basmati rice or chapatis, to serve

Takes 20 minutes • Serves 4

1 Heat the oil in a frying pan, then fry the onions over a medium heat until soft and beginning to brown, for about 5 minutes. Meanwhile, reserve 8 of the tomato wedges, then whiz the remainder in a food processor with the ginger and garlic.

2 Add the curry paste to the pan for around 30 seconds. Stir through the tomato mix and remaining tomato wedges, then bubble over a high heat for 5 minutes, stirring so the sauce doesn't catch. Mix in the prawns and peas; simmer until the prawns are pink and cooked through. Scatter with coriander, then serve with rice or chapatis.

• Per serving 236 kcalories, protein 24g, carbohydrate 18g, fat 8g, saturated fat 1g, fibre 6g, sugar 10g, salt 1.24g

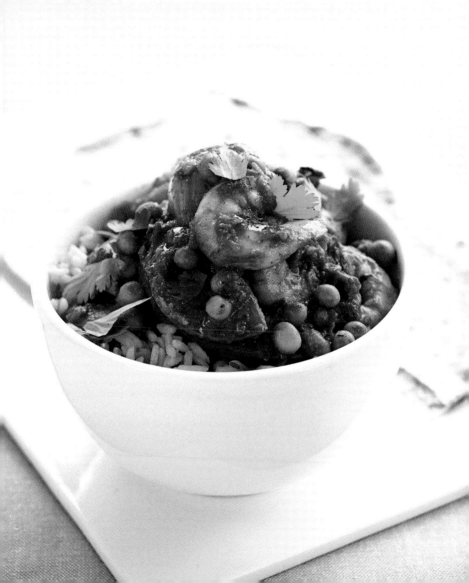

When using bottled passata or canned tomatoes, try adding a pinch of sugar – it will help to bring out the natural sweetness of the tomatoes.

White fish with spicy beans and chorizo

1 tbsp olive oil
1 onion, chopped
1 small rosemary sprig, leaves finely chopped
25g/1oz chorizo or other spicy sausage, chopped
2 fat garlic cloves, crushed
700g bottle passata
410g can cannellini beans in water, drained and rinsed
200g/8oz shredded green cabbage
a pinch of sugar
4 × skinless chunky haddock or cod fillets
crusty bread, to serve

Takes 20 minutes • Serves 4

1 Heat the oil in a large frying pan, then soften the onion for 5 minutes. Add the rosemary, chorizo and garlic, then fry for 2 minutes more until the chorizo is starting to crisp. Tip in the passata, beans, cabbage and sugar, season, then simmer for 5 minutes.

2 Add the fish to the pan, leaving the tops of the fillets peeking out of the sauce, then cover with a lid and leave to cook for 3–5 minutes or until the flesh flakes easily. Delicious served with crusty bread.

• Per serving 304 kcalories, protein 36g, carbohydrate 27g, fat 6g, saturated fat 1g, fibre 6g, sugar 11g, salt 1.23g

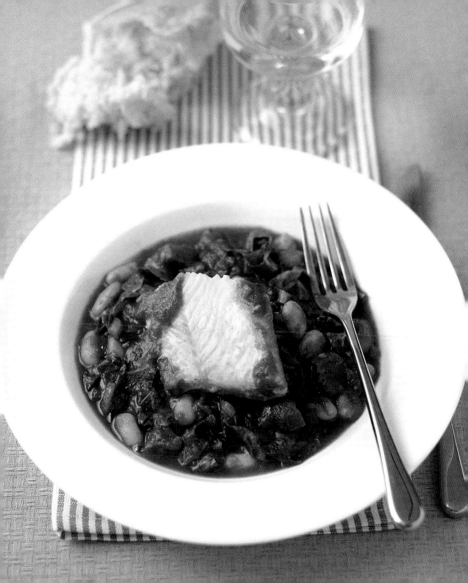

With a flavour and look of the sunny Med, this wonderful one-pot can be on the table in just 20 minutes. It's a healthy choice too, because it counts as two of your 5-a-day.

Spanish rice and prawn one-pot

1 onion, sliced
1 red and 1 green pepper, seeded and sliced
50g/2oz chorizo, sliced
2 garlic cloves, crushed
1 tbsp olive oil
250g/9oz easy-cook basmati rice
400g can chopped tomatoes
200g/8oz raw peeled prawns, (defrosted if frozen)

Takes 20 minutes • Serves 4

1 Boil the kettle. In a non-stick frying or shallow pan with a lid, fry the onion, peppers, chorizo and garlic in the oil over a high heat for 3 minutes. Stir in the rice and chopped tomatoes with 500ml/18fl oz boiling water, cover, then cook over a high heat for 12 minutes.

2 Uncover, then stir – the rice should be almost tender. Stir in the prawns, with a splash more water if the rice is looking dry, then cook for another minute until the prawns are just pink and the rice is tender. Serve at the table, straight from the pot.

• Per serving 356 kcalories, protein 19g, carbohydrate 59g, fat 7g, saturated fat 2g, fibre 4g, sugar 7g, salt 0.85g

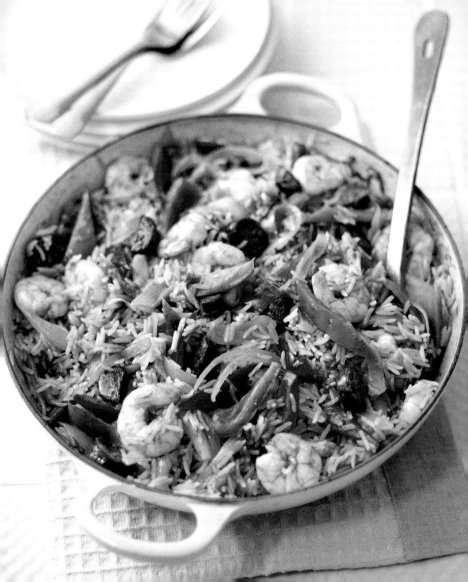

You can also make this chowder with fish – cut 300g/10oz skinned smoked haddock or cod into chunks and add at the same time as the peas and sweetcorn, replacing the chicken and ham.

Chunky chicken & ham chowder

1 tbsp sunflower oil
2 leeks, thinly sliced
3 medium potatoes, peeled and cut into small cubes
1 tbsp plain flour
700ml/1¼ pints skimmed milk
2 ready-roasted chicken breasts, skin removed and cut into chunks
2 thick slices ham, chopped
175g/6oz each frozen sweetcorn and frozen peas

Takes 30 minutes • Serves 4

1 Heat the oil in a large pan and fry the leeks over a low heat for 3 minutes until softened. Stir in the potatoes and flour, then slowly blend in the milk, stirring with a wooden spoon. Bring to the boil and simmer, uncovered, for 10-12 minutes until the potatoes are soft.
2 Add the chicken, ham, sweetcorn and peas, then stir over a medium heat for 5 minutes or until hot and bubbling. Season to taste and serve with crusty bread.

• Per serving 341 kcalories, protein 34g, carbohydrate 37g, fat 7g, saturated fat 2g, fibre 5g, sugar 12g, salt 0.66g

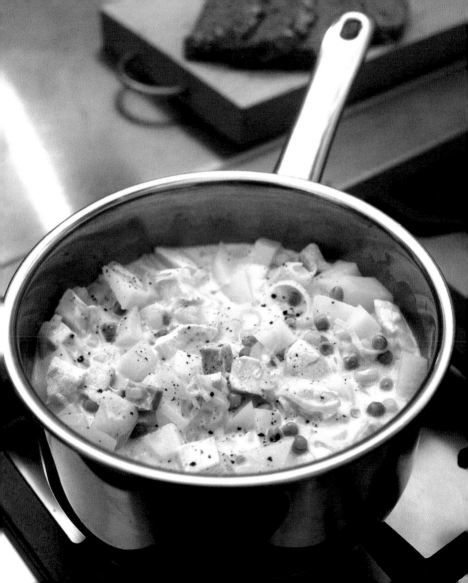

The dried mushrooms give a real depth of flavour to this dish. Keep a pack in the storecupboard and this will be a supper you can always rustle up in half an hour.

Baked porcini and thyme risotto

25g pack dried porcini mushrooms
2 tbsp olive oil
1 small onion, finely chopped
2 garlic cloves, crushed
2 tsp thyme leaves, plus extra to garnish
350g/12oz risotto rice
750ml/1¼ pints hot vegetable stock
100ml/3½fl oz white wine
a handful of grated Parmesan, plus shavings, to garnish

Takes 30 minutes • Serves 4

1 Put the mushrooms in a bowl, pour over 425ml/14fl oz boiling water and leave to soak for 10 minutes. Meanwhile, heat the oil in an ovenproof pan and fry the onion for 2 minutes until starting to soften. Add the garlic and cook for another minute.

2 Preheat the oven to 190°C/170°C fan/gas 5. Drain the mushrooms, reserving the liquid, and chop. Add the mushrooms, thyme and rice to the pan, then stir well. Strain over the mushroom liquid, pour in the stock and wine, and bring to the boil.

3 Season to taste, cover and bake for 25 minutes or until the rice is just cooked and all the liquid has been absorbed. Stir in the grated Parmesan, check the seasoning and sprinkle with extra thyme leaves and Parmesan shavings to serve.

• Per serving 374 kcalories, protein 9g, carbohydrate 75g, fat 6g, saturated fat 1g, fibre 2g, sugar 5g, salt 0.64g

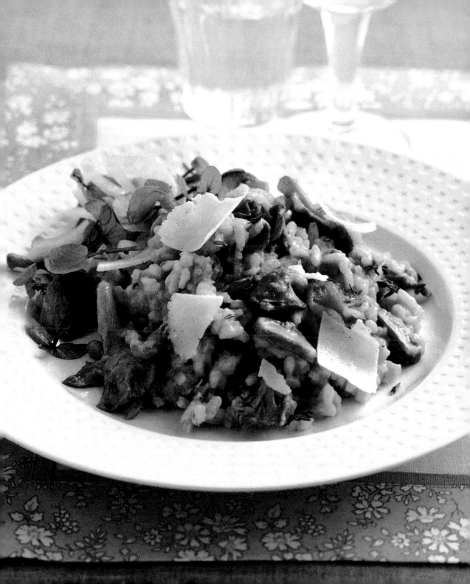

Courgette slices or broccoli florets can be used instead of the French
beans for a change in this healthy casserole for two.

All-in-one chicken, squash
& new potato casserole

¼ small butternut squash, peeled,
seeded and diced
(200g/8oz approx)
8 small new potatoes
1 tsp ground coriander
1 tbsp thyme leaves
600ml/1pt chicken stock
1 garlic clove, crushed
2 skinless chicken breasts
175g/6oz prepared French beans
25g/1oz pitted green olives in brine,
drained

Takes 45 minutes • Serves 2

1 Preheat the oven to 190°C/170°C fan/
gas 5. Put the butternut squash, potatoes,
ground coriander, thyme, stock and garlic into
a flameproof casserole. Season and bring to
the boil, then simmer gently for 10 minutes.
2 Tuck in the chicken breasts, making sure
that they are submerged. Cover and transfer
to the oven for 15 minutes until the chicken
is cooked through. Lift out the chicken and
vegetables, set aside and keep warm, then
boil the stock on the hob until reduced by
half. Add the beans and olives, simmer until
cooked. Season and serve.

• Per serving 413 kcalories, protein 41g, carbohydrate
50g, fat 6.5g, saturated fat 1.5g, fibre 8g, sugar 13g,
salt 1g

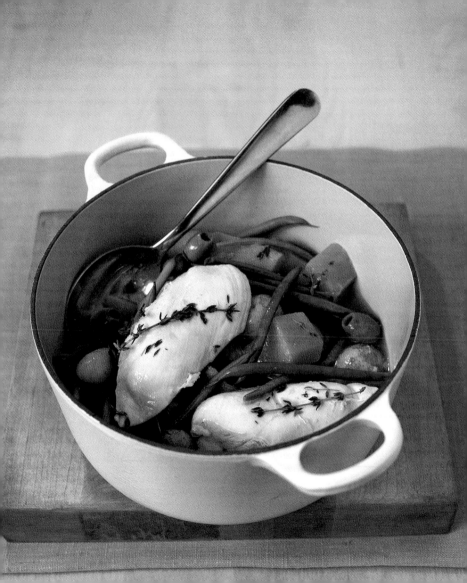

Bubbling and golden brown straight from the oven, moussaka is always a firm favourite, and this one has all of your 5-a-day in just one portion.

Roast veggie moussaka with feta

2 yellow peppers, seeded and cut into chunks
2 red onions, cut into wedges
2 medium courgettes, thickly sliced
1 large aubergine, cut into chunks
1 tbsp olive oil
85g/3oz feta
1 egg
200ml pot Greek yogurt
700g bottle passata
2 tbsp chopped fresh oregano or 2 tsp dried
crusty bread, to serve

Takes 55 minutes • Serves 4

1 Preheat the oven to 200°C/180°C fan/gas 6. Scatter the vegetables in a large roasting tin. Toss with the oil, season, then roast for 25 minutes until softened.
2 Break up the feta in a small bowl with a fork, then mix well with the egg, yogurt and seasoning. When the vegetables are ready, tip them into an ovenproof dish, then stir in the passata and oregano. Spoon over the creamy feta topping, turn up the oven to 220°C/200°C fan/gas 7, then bake for around 20–25 minutes until the filling is hot and the topping is beginning to brown and bubble. Serve the moussaka with crusty bread.

• Per serving 223 kcalories, protein 11g, carbohydrate 24g, fat 10g, saturated fat 4g, fibre 5g, sugar 17g, salt 1.74g

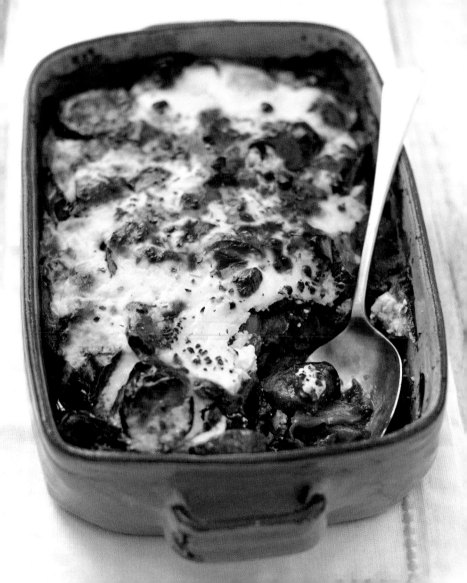

Make your own pizza and you can tailor it to your choice – this one is low-fat, low cost, meat free and truly delicious.

Butternut and rosemary pizza

500g pack white bread mix
flour, for rolling
1 tbsp olive oil, plus extra
to drizzle (optional)
1 large butternut squash, peeled,
seeded and cut into small cubes
2 red onions, sliced
3 rosemary sprigs, leaves chopped,
plus extra small sprigs to garnish
1 tbsp caster sugar
2 tbsp balsamic vinegar
100g/4oz feta
salad, to serve

Takes 45 minutes • Serves 4–6

1 Make the bread dough according to the packet instructions, knead for a few minutes, then, using flour to prevent sticking, roll into two large rounds and lift on to baking sheets.
2 Heat the oil in a large frying pan, then fry the squash with the onions and chopped rosemary for 5 minutes until beginning to soften and brown. Splash in about 200ml/7fl oz water, then cook over a fierce heat for 10 minutes, stirring until the squash is tender and almost all the liquid has gone. Preheat the oven to 220°C/200°C fan/gas 7.
3 Stir the sugar, vinegar and some seasoning into the squash mix, then spread over the pizza dough. Top with a few small rosemary sprigs, crumble over the feta, then drizzle with a little more oil, if you like. Bake one at a time for 15 minutes until the pizzas are golden and crisp. Serve with salad.

• Per serving (4) 630 kcalories, protein 24g, carbohydrate 115g, fat 11g, saturated fat 4g, fibre 9g, sugar 20g, salt 2.92g

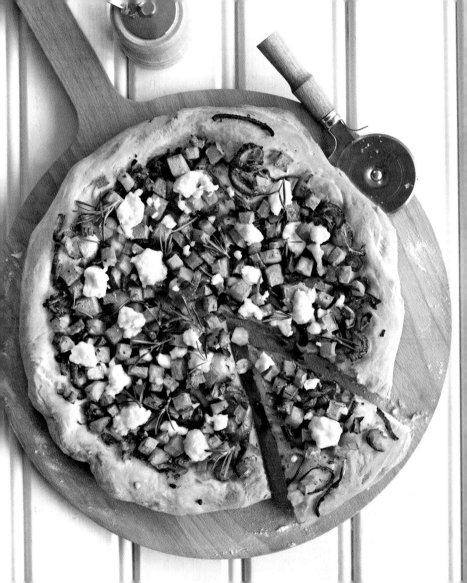

These make peppers a light and colourful lunch or supper. Packed with goodness, this dish counts as three of your 5-a-day.

Gremolata couscous-stuffed peppers

85g/3oz couscous
2 tbsp raisins
50ml/2fl oz hot vegetable stock
1 tsp clear honey
zest and juice of 1 lemon
2 garlic cloves
1 small bunch flatleaf parsley
150ml pot low-fat natural yogurt
2 tomatoes, roughly chopped
2 red peppers, halved and seeded
1 tbsp olive oil
simple green salad, to serve

Takes 55 minutes • Serves 2

1 Preheat the oven to 190°C/170°C fan/ gas 5. Put the couscous and raisins in a heatproof bowl. Stir together the stock, honey and lemon juice, then pour over the couscous. Cover and leave to absorb for 5 minutes.

2 Meanwhile, make the gremolata. Put the lemon zest, garlic and parsley in a mini food processor, then whiz until fine (or finely chop everything together). Stir 1 tablespoon of this mixture into the yogurt, then set aside. Stir the remaining mixture into the couscous with the tomatoes and some seasoning.

3 Spoon the couscous mixture into each pepper half, then sit them in a small roasting tin. Drizzle with oil, then bake for 40 minutes until the peppers are tender. Serve with the yogurt and a simple green salad on the side.

• Per serving 302 kcalories, protein 9g, carbohydrate 52g, fat 8g, saturated fat 1g, fibre 4g, sugar 30g, salt 0.23g

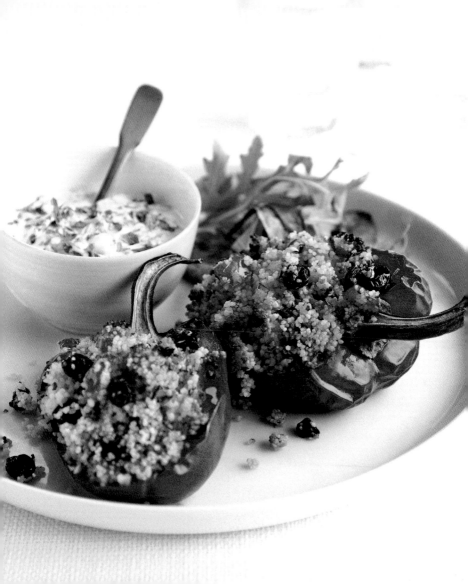

An exciting new idea for a salad that can be served as a main meal. The delicious sesame dressing adds zing to the vibrant veg.

Puy lentil salad with soy beans, sugar snaps and broccoli

200g/8oz Puy lentils
1 litre/1¾ pints hot vegetable stock
200g/8oz Tenderstem broccoli
140g/5oz frozen soy beans, thawed
140g/5oz sugar snap peas
1 red chilli, seeded and sliced

FOR THE DRESSING
2 tbsp sesame oil
juice of 1 lemon
1 garlic clove, chopped
2½ tbsp reduced-salt soy sauce
3cm knob of ginger, finely grated
1 tbsp clear honey

Takes 25 minutes • Serves 4

1 Boil the lentils in the stock for about 15 minutes until just cooked. Drain, then tip into a large bowl. Bring a pan of salted water to the boil, throw in the broccoli for 1 minute, add the beans and peas for 1 minute more. Drain, then cool under cold water. Pat dry, then add to the bowl with the lentils.
2 Mix together the dressing ingredients with some seasoning. Pour over the lentils and vegetables, then mix in well with the sliced chilli. Pile on to a serving platter or divide among four plates and serve.

• Per serving 302 kcalories, protein 22g, carbohydrate 42g, fat 7g, saturated fat 1g, fibre 8g, sugar 9g, salt 1.41g

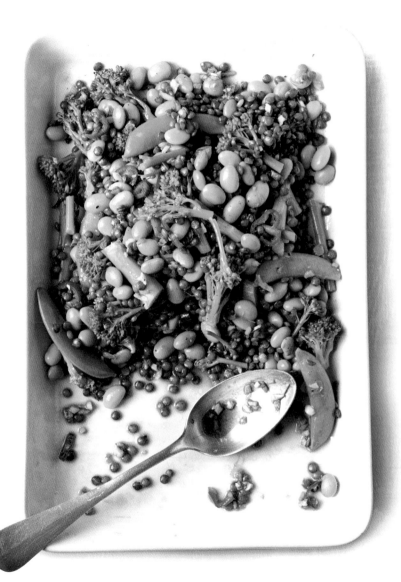

The pine nuts add a nice toasty crunch to this
meal in a bowl. You can ring the changes by using
tomatoes instead of the mushrooms.

Vitality veggie pasta

250g pack pappardelle pasta
1 small butternut squash, peeled,
seeded and chopped
into chunks
2 tbsp olive oil
a small handful of pine nuts
1 plump garlic clove, finely chopped
4 large field mushrooms, sliced
250g bag spinach leaves
grated Parmesan and chilli flakes,
to serve (optional)

Takes 25 minutes • Serves 4

1 Cook the pasta according to the packet
instructions. When the pasta has 5 minutes
left to cook, tip in the squash and cook with
the pasta for the remaining time.
2 Meanwhile, heat half the oil in a large
frying pan. Sizzle the pine nuts until they
start to colour, stir in the garlic and cook for
a moment just to soften. Add the remaining
oil, turn up the heat, add the mushrooms and
cook for 2–3 minutes until they start to soften.
Turn the heat to maximum, add the spinach
to the pan and cook for 1–2 minutes until
completely wilted.
3 Drain the pasta and squash, then mix in
with the vegetables until everything is nicely
combined and serve. You could also pass
round grated Parmesan and chilli flakes, if
people want them.

• Per serving 377 kcalories, protein 13g, carbohydrate
62g, fat 10g, saturated fat 1g, fibre 7g, added sugar
none, salt 0.27g

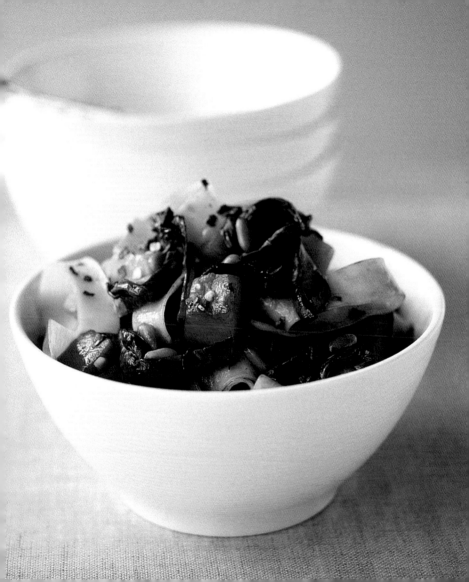

A golden pasta bake is always a popular choice with the family.
The only accompaniment you need is a crisp green salad
and some crusty bread.

Easy oven frittata

½ tsp olive oil
85g/3oz fusilli or macaroni
1 leek or 1 bunch spring onions, chopped
85g/3oz frozen or canned sweetcorn
85g/3oz frozen peas
1 red pepper, seeded and chopped
2 large eggs
150ml/¼ pint semi-skimmed milk
1 tbsp thyme leaves (preferably lemon thyme)
50g/2oz extra-mature Cheddar, grated
2 tbsp finely grated Parmesan

Takes 1 hour • Serves 4

1 Preheat the oven to 190°C/170°C fan/gas 5. Grease a 1.2-litre/2-pint baking dish with the olive oil.
2 Cook the pasta in salted boiling water in a large pan for 8 minutes. Add all the vegetables and cook for another 2–3 minutes until the pasta is tender and the vegetables slightly softened. Drain, then tip into the baking dish and mix well.
3 Beat together the eggs and milk in a jug, and add the thyme. Mix the two cheeses together and add most of it to the egg mixture, then season. Pour into the baking dish, mix gently, then scatter the rest of the cheese on top. Bake for 35–40 minutes until set and golden. Cool for just a few minutes, then serve.

• Per serving 277 kcalories, protein 16g, carbohydrate 29g, fat 12g, saturated fat 6g, fibre 3g, sugar 2g, salt 0.7g

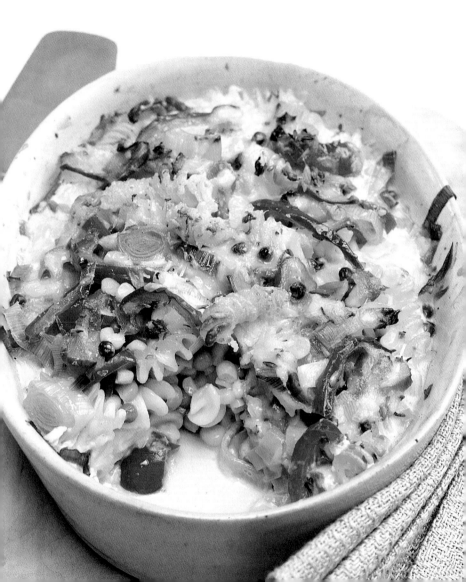

The secret to keeping down the fat content is to use low-fat halloumi cheese bulked out with plenty of vegetables.

Halloumi kebabs with thyme and lemon baste

2 medium courgettes
1 large red onion
250g/9oz low-fat halloumi, cut into 16 chunks
16 cherry tomatoes
warm pitta bread, to serve

FOR THE LEMON BASTE
1 tbsp olive oil
2 tbsp fresh lemon juice
2 tsp thyme leaves (preferably lemon thyme)
1 tsp Dijon mustard

Takes 25 minutes • Serves 4

1 Halve the courgettes lengthways, then thickly slice. Cut the onion into wedges and separate into pieces. Thread the halloumi, cherry tomatoes, courgettes and onion on to eight skewers. Cover and chill the kebabs until you are ready to cook.

2 To make the baste, mix together the olive oil, lemon juice, thyme, mustard and a little seasoning, to taste.

3 Preheat the barbecue or grill and arrange the kebabs on the rack. Brush with the baste, stirring it first to make sure the ingredients are blended. Cook for 4–5 minutes, turning often, until the cheese begins to turn golden and the vegetables are just tender. Serve while still hot with warm pitta bread.

• Per serving 194 kcalories, protein 17g, carbohydrate 7g, fat 11g, saturated fat 5g, fibre 1g, sugar 0g, salt 2.4g

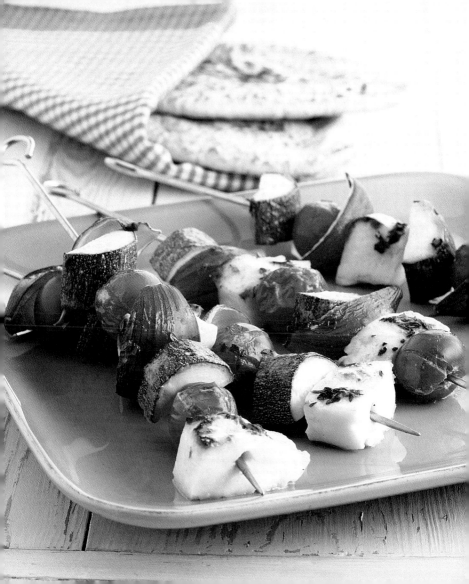

This soft, delicious low-fat risotto makes the most of the summer's fresh produce. It's a great way to get kids to eat their vegetables, especially if you grate over a little cheese.

Summer courgette risotto

1 tbsp olive oil
1 onion, finely chopped
2 garlic cloves, finely chopped
3 ripe tomatoes, roughly chopped
350g/12oz carnaroli or other risotto rice
1 tsp chopped rosemary
1.5 litres/2¾ pints hot vegetable stock
3 courgettes, finely diced
140g/5oz peas, fresh or frozen
a large handful of basil leaves, lightly torn

Takes 45 minutes • Serves 4

1 Heat the oil in a large pan. Cook the onion and garlic for 5 minutes until the onion has softened. Add the tomatoes and cook for 3–4 minutes until softened and pulpy, then add the rice and rosemary.

2 Pour in half the stock and leave to cook for 10 minutes or until the liquid has evaporated, stirring from time to time. Add the rest of the stock, then continue to cook for a further 5 minutes.

3 Stir in the courgettes and peas, then cook for another 5 minutes or so, stirring until the rice is tender but the mixture is still a bit saucy. Season with plenty of black pepper, then add the basil and stir until wilted. Serve immediately.

• Per serving 406 kcalories, protein 14g, carbohydrate 82g, fat 5g, saturated fat 1g, fibre 7g, sugar 9g, salt 0.51g

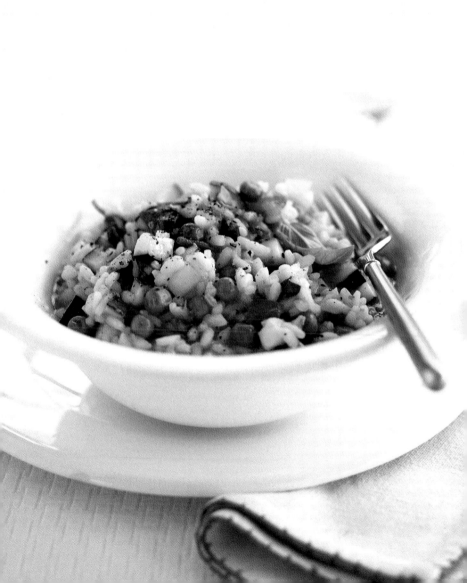

This Indian-inspired rice stuffing can also be used in large beefsteak tomatoes, but they will take less time to cook than the peppers – roast for just 20 minutes without adding the water or foil.

Biryani-stuffed peppers

4 tbsp olive oil
1 onion, chopped
2 garlic cloves, chopped
1 cinnamon stick
1 tsp each ground turmeric, ground cumin, ground coriander, cardamom pods
250g/9oz basmati rice
a handful of parsley leaves, roughly chopped
a handful of coriander leaves, roughly chopped
zest and juice of 1 lemon
50g/2oz each pine nuts and raisins
6 red peppers

Takes 1¼ hours • Serves 6

1 Preheat the oven to 200°C/180°C fan/gas 6. Heat half the oil in a pan and fry the onion and garlic. Add the spices and cook for a few minutes more. Stir the rice through. Cover the rice with water, put a lid on the pan and bring to the boil. Turn down the heat and simmer for 10 minutes until just cooked. Stir the herbs, lemon zest and juice, pine nuts and raisins through the rice.
2 Cut around the stalks of the peppers and discard. Use a teaspoon to scrape out the pith and seeds. Stuff the peppers with the rice and sit them in a small roasting tin. Pour 100ml/3½fl oz water into the tin and drizzle with the remaining oil. Cover the tin with foil, then roast for 20 minutes. Remove the foil, then continue to cook for 20 minutes until the peppers are soft and just starting to fall apart.

• Per serving 274 kcalories, protein 6g, carbohydrate 46g, fat 9g, saturated fat 1g, fibre 3g, sugar 11g, salt 0.02g

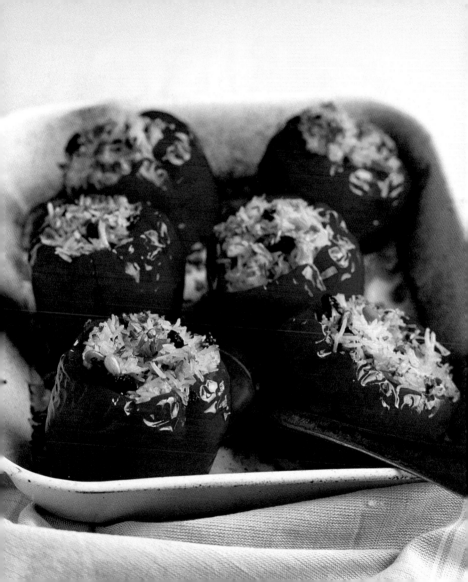

To make a creamy version of this quick pasta dish, simply stir in 100g/3½oz ricotta with the cooked mushrooms.

Herby mushroom pasta

250g/9oz field or portobello mushrooms, thickly sliced
2 tsp wholegrain mustard
3 garlic cloves, sliced or crushed
150ml/¼ pint vegetable stock (from a cube is fine)
200g/8oz penne pasta (or other tube shapes)
3 tbsp flatleaf parsley, chopped
zest of 1 lemon

Takes 20 minutes • Serves 2

1 Put the mushrooms, mustard, garlic and vegetable stock into a frying pan, bring to the boil and simmer for 5 minutes or until the stock has nearly all evaporated and the mushrooms are soft.
2 Meanwhile, cook the pasta according to the packet instructions. Drain and toss with the mushrooms, parsley and lemon zest. Season to taste and serve straight away.

• Per serving 235 kcalories, protein 9g, carbohydrate 49g, fat 2g, saturated fat 0.2g, fibre 3g, sugar 2g, salt 0.25g

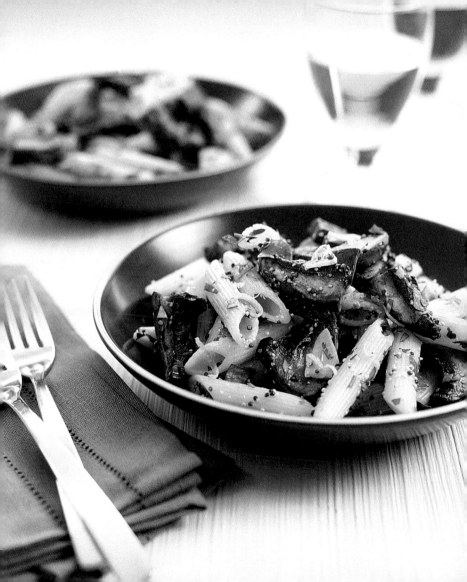

This healthier version of spag bol is made with a mix of tasty vegetables and lentils, with oregano and cinnamon adding a good flavour. Make double and freeze a meal for another day.

Veggie spag bol

1 onion
1 carrot
1 stick celery
1 red pepper
2 tbsp olive oil
100g/4oz red lentils
400g can tomatoes
600ml/1 pint vegetable stock
2 tsp dried oregano
½ tsp ground cinnamon
350g/12oz spaghetti
freshly grated Parmesan, to serve

Takes 40 minutes • Serves 4

1 Roughly chop the vegetables then whiz them in a food processor until finely chopped.
2 Heat the oil in a large pan and fry the vegetables for about 8 minutes until soft. Stir in the lentils, tomatoes, stock, oregano and cinnamon. Bring to the boil, reduce the heat, cover and simmer for 20 minutes. Season then simmer for a further 5 minutes.
3 Cook the spaghetti according to the packet instructions. Serve with the sauce and grated cheese.

• Per serving 484 kcalories, protein 19g, carbohydrate 90g, fat 8g, saturated fat 1g, fibre 6g, sugar none, salt 0.66g

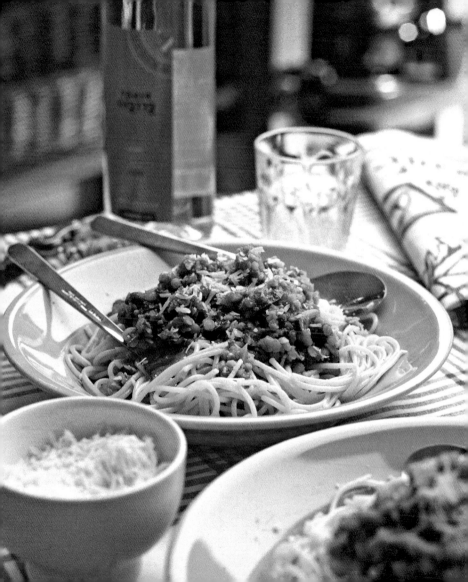

By using low-fat mozzarella, just a little olive oil and plenty of vegetables, a pizza can make a healthy meal!

Roasted spring vegetable pizza

200g/8oz strong plain flour
½ tsp salt
1 tsp easy-blend dried yeast
150ml/¼ pint warm water
olive oil, for brushing

FOR THE TOPPING
2 red peppers
1 leek
1 tsp olive oil
4 tbsp passata
125g pack light mozzarella
12 cherry tomatoes
3 tbsp frozen peas
2 tbsp freshly grated Parmesan

Takes 1 hour • Serves 4

1 Preheat the oven to 220°C/200°C fan/gas 7. Tip the flour, salt and yeast into a bowl and mix well. Add the warm water and mix to a soft dough. Knead for 2–3 minutes, then roll out to a 30-cm round. Brush a large baking sheet with a thin slick of oil, then add the pizza base. Cover with a clean tea towel.
2 Cut the peppers into rings and slice the leek. Toss the leek and red peppers in the oil and season with salt and pepper. Spread over a baking sheet and roast for 10 minutes.
3 Spread the pizza base with the passata. Scatter over the leek and red pepper. Thinly slice the mozzarella and arrange over the vegetables. Scatter over the whole cherry tomatoes and peas and sprinkle with the parmesan. Bake for 15–20 minutes, until the crust is crisp and lightly browned.

• Per serving 290 kcalories, protein 15g carbohydrate 47g, fat 6g, saturated fat 3g, fibre 4g, added sugar none, salt 0.84g

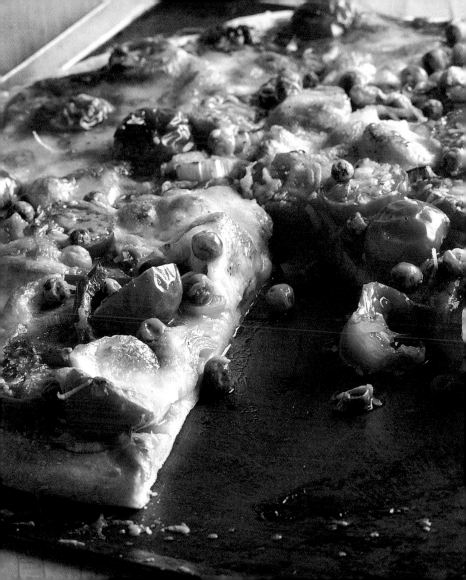

Just five ingredients make a terrific-tasting risotto
that's easy to cook in the microwave. The squash adds
a sweetness to this ultimate comfort food.

Microwave butternut squash risotto

250g/9oz risotto rice
700ml/1¼ pint hot vegetable stock
1 medium butternut squash
a big handful of grated Parmesan,
plus extra to garnish
a handful of sage leaves, roughly
chopped

Takes 25 minutes • Serves 4

1 Tip the rice into a large bowl, then add
500ml/18fl oz of the hot vegetable stock.
Cover with cling film and microwave on
High for 5 minutes.
2 Meanwhile, peel and seed the squash
then cut into medium chunks. Stir the
rice, then add the squash and the rest of
the stock. Re-cover with cling film, then
microwave for another 15 minutes, stirring
halfway, until almost all the stock is absorbed
and the rice and squash are tender.
3 Leave the risotto to sit for 2 minutes, then
stir in the cheese and sage leaves. Serve
topped with more grated Parmesan.

• Per serving 313 kcalories, protein 10g, carbohydrate
66g, fat 3g, saturated fat 1g, fibre 4g, sugar 9g,
salt 1.04g

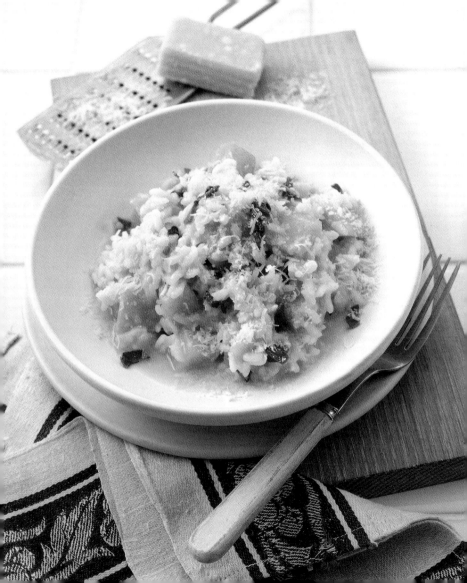

The fresh, simple flavours of lemon and mint work perfectly together for a light full-of-summer lunch that's low in fat.

Spring-into-summer pasta

350g/12oz tagliatelle
500g/1lb 2oz courgettes
190g pack shelled fresh peas,
or use frozen
zest and juice of 1 lemon
a handful of mint leaves, chopped
250g pot ricotta

Takes 15 minutes • Serves 4

1 Cook the tagliatelle according to the packet instructions.
2 Meanwhile, cut the courgettes into thin finger-length sticks. When the pasta has 2 minutes left to cook, tip the courgettes and peas into the pan, then cook until just tender. Drain and return to the pan.
3 Toss in the lemon juice, zest and most of the mint, then season to taste. Divide among four bowls, spoon small dollops of ricotta over each and sprinkle with the remaining mint.

• Per serving 457 kcalories, protein 22g, carbohydrate 75g, fat 10g, saturated fat 5g, fibre 6g, sugar none, salt 0.19g

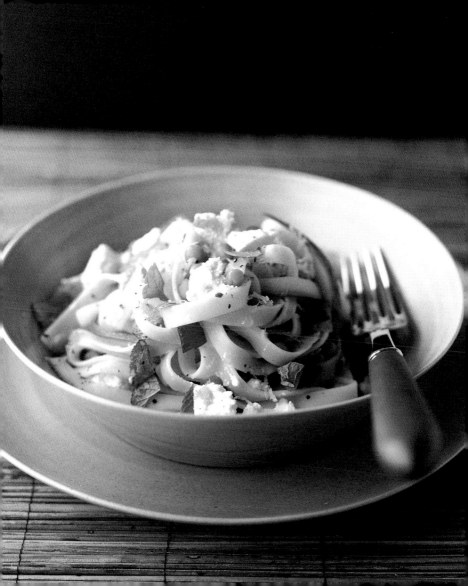

Serve this dish at room temperature with a Greek salad and crusty bread for a light lunch, or on top of some toasted sourdough as a snack.

Greek baked beans

400g/14oz dried butter beans
3 tbsp Greek extra-virgin olive oil, plus extra to drizzle
1 Spanish onion, finely chopped
2 garlic cloves, finely chopped
2 tbsp tomato purée
800g/1lb 12oz ripe tomatoes, skinned and roughly chopped
1 tsp sugar
1 tsp dried oregano
a pinch of ground cinnamon
2 tbsp chopped flat-leaf parsley, plus extra to garnish

Takes 2 hours 20 minutes, plus overnight soaking • Serves 4

1 Soak the beans overnight in plenty of water. Drain, rinse, then place in a pan covered with water. Bring to the boil, reduce the heat, then simmer for about 50 minutes until tender but not soft. Drain, then set aside.
2 Preheat the oven to 180°C/160°C fan/gas 4. Heat the olive oil in a large frying pan, tip in the onion and garlic, then cook over a medium heat for 10 minutes until softened. Add the tomato purée, cook for 1 minute, add remaining ingredients, then simmer for 2–3 minutes. Season, then stir in the beans.
3 Tip into a large ovenproof dish, then bake for 1 hour, uncovered and without stirring, until the beans are tender. The beans will absorb all the fabulous flavours and the sauce will thicken. Allow to cool, then scatter with parsley and drizzle with a little oil to serve.

• Per serving 431 kcalories, protein 22g, carbohydrate 66g, fat 11g, saturated fat 1g, fibre 19g, sugar 15g, salt 0.2g

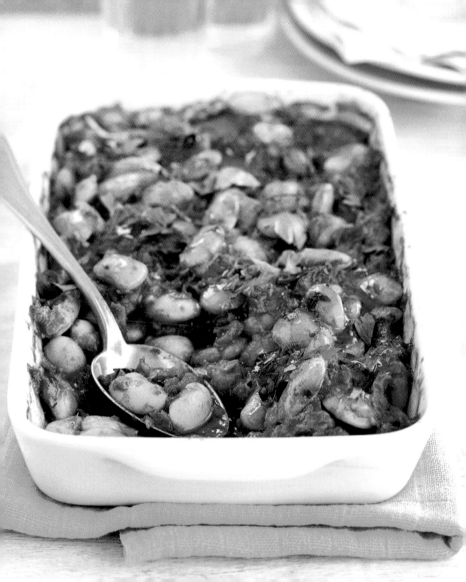

Using a ready-made curry paste means you have all the authentic flavour without having to buy a long list of spices.

Sweet & hot vegetable curry

1 tbsp sunflower oil
3 tbsp Vindaloo curry paste
1 tbsp soft brown sugar
juice of ½ lemon
2 courgettes, thickly sliced
300g/10oz cauliflower florets (about ½ a head)
400ml/14fl oz passata
400g can chickpeas, drained and rinsed
250g bag spinach leaves
basmati rice, to serve

Takes 35 minutes • Serves 6

1 Heat the oil in a large pan, add the curry paste and fry for 1 minute. Add the sugar and lemon juice, cook for 1 minute, then tip in the courgettes and cauliflower, and cook for 2 minutes. Now stir in the passata, plus 100ml/3½fl oz water and the chickpeas, and season to taste. Bring to the boil, cover with a lid and simmer for 15 minutes.
2 Just before serving, throw in the spinach, give it a stir and remove from the heat once the leaves have just wilted. Serve with boiled basmati rice.

• Per serving 142 kcalories, protein 8g, carbohydrate 16g, fat 6g, saturated fat none, fibre 4g, sugar 8g, salt 1.01g

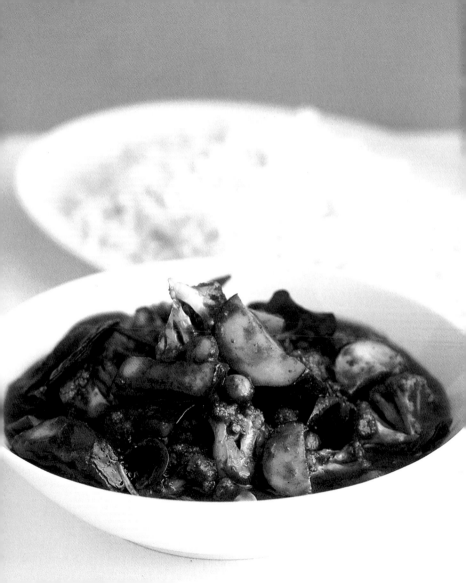

An attractive and quick way of serving lasagne. The bean mixture is simply stacked with the cooked lasagne sheets on individual plates.

Chilli bean open lasagne

1 tbsp olive oil
1 onion, chopped
2 garlic cloves, crushed
1 red chilli, seeded and finely sliced
1 small aubergine, chopped
1 large courgette, chopped
410g can borlotti beans, drained and rinsed
400g can chopped tomatoes
2 tbsp tomato purée
250g packet fresh lasagne sheets
a handful of basil leaves, torn, plus extra to garnish
100g/4oz Cheddar, grated

Takes 30 minutes • Serves 4

1 Heat the oil, then fry the onion for around 2–3 minutes. Add the garlic, chilli, aubergine and courgette, then fry for a further 2–3 minutes. Stir in the beans, tomatoes, purée and some seasoning. Bring to the boil, then simmer for 5 minutes.

2 Meanwhile, cook the lasagne according to the packet instructions. Drain, then halve each sheet diagonally. Stir the torn basil leaves into the beans.

3 Place a spoonful of the mixture on each of four warmed serving plates, and top each with a quarter of the lasagne triangles. Top with the remaining bean mixture and a quarter of the cheese per plate. Garnish with the extra basil.

• Per serving 400 kcalories, protein 17g, carbohydrate 73g, fat 6g, saturated fat 1g, fibre 11g, sugar none, salt 1.21g

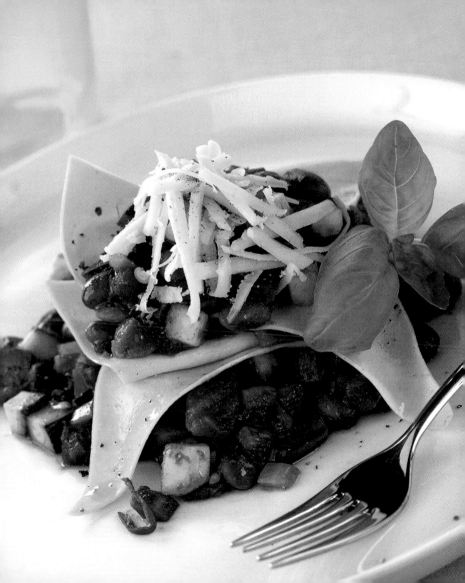

Sweet potatoes can become waterlogged when boiled,
so mash them over a low heat and any excess water
will evaporate, leaving fluffy spuds.

Moroccan spiced fish with ginger mash

2 large sweet potatoes, peeled and
cut into chunks
2 tsp butter, softened
1 garlic clove, crushed
½–1 tsp harissa paste
zest of 1 lemon
a small handful of coriander,
chopped
fingertip-size knob of ginger,
finely grated
2 skinless white fish fillets
green veg, to serve

Takes 30 minutes • Serves 2

1 Preheat the oven to 200°C/180°C fan/
gas 6. Cook the sweet potatoes in boiling
salted water for about 10 minutes or until
just tender when pierced with a knife.
2 Meanwhile, mix together the butter with
the garlic, harissa, lemon zest, chopped
coriander and some seasoning. Set aside.
3 When the potatoes are ready, drain
thoroughly and mash with the ginger and
seasoning, then keep warm.
4 Put the fish in a roasting tin, season,
then spread half the flavoured butter over
each fillet. Roast for about 8 minutes until
just cooked through. Serve with the ginger
mash and some green veg.

• Per serving 445 kcalories, protein 36g, carbohydrate
65g, fat 7g, saturated fat 3g, fibre 7g, sugar 17g,
salt 0.67g

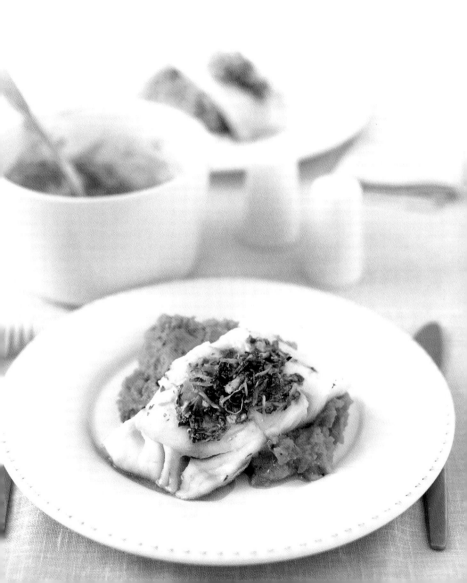

This pork is wonderful with some plain boiled rice and steamed greens. The pork can be tossed in the marinade just before cooking or marinated overnight.

Sticky pork

500g/1lb 2oz piece pork fillet
rice and steamed greens, to serve

FOR THE MARINADE
4 tbsp soy sauce
1 tbsp clear honey
finely grated zest and juice of
1 orange
large knob of ginger,
finely grated

Takes 35 minutes • Serves 4

1 Tip all the marinade ingredients into a shallow dish and stir to combine. Coat the pork in the marinade and, if you have time, leave for 1 hour or, even better, overnight.
2 Preheat the oven to 200°C/180°C fan/ gas 6. Heat an ovenproof pan and take the pork out of the marinade. Brown in the pan on all sides, then baste over the rest of the marinade and roast the pork in the oven for 20 minutes until cooked all the way through, basting with its juices every 5 minutes or so. Serve the pork sliced with rice and your favourite steamed greens.

• Per serving 165 kcalories, protein 28g, carbohydrate 3g, fat 5g, saturated fat 2g, fibre none, sugar 3g, salt 1.56g

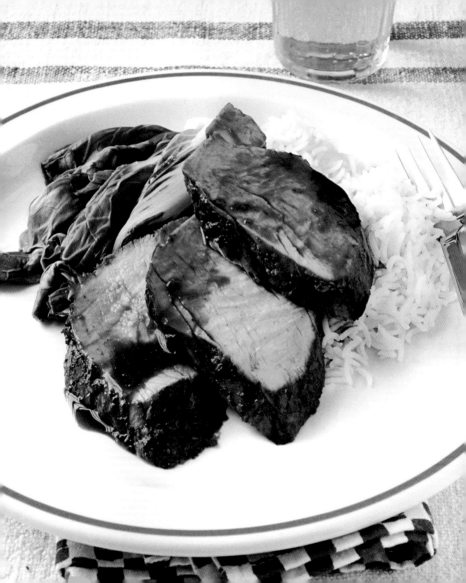

Perfect for a Saturday-night supper with the family.
The children will love the crispy-coated chicken and zesty dip.

Sesame chicken with soy dip

140g/5oz breadcrumbs
3 tbsp sesame seeds
1 tsp Chinese five-spice
4 skinless chicken breasts,
flattened a little
1 egg, lightly beaten
300g/10oz Tenderstem broccoli
3 tbsp soy sauce
juice of 1 lemon
juice of 1 lime, plus extra wedges
to serve
1 tbsp caster sugar

Takes 35 minutes • Serves 4

1 Preheat the oven to 200°C/180°C fan/
gas 6 and line a baking sheet with baking
parchment. Mix the breadcrumbs, sesame
seeds, five-spice and a little seasoning on a
plate. Pat dry the chicken, dip into the egg,
then roll in the breadcrumb mix. Arrange
on the baking sheet, then bake for 25–30
minutes until crisp and cooked through.
2 When the chicken is almost ready, cook
the broccoli in salted water for a few minutes
until just tender. Mix the soy sauce with the
citrus juices and sugar to make a dipping
sauce. Serve the crispy chicken with the
broccoli and little dishes of the sauce for
dipping, plus lime wedges for squeezing over.

• Per serving 398 kcalories, protein 44g, carbohydrate
34g, fat 10g, saturated fat 2g, fibre 4g, sugar 8g,
salt 3.01g

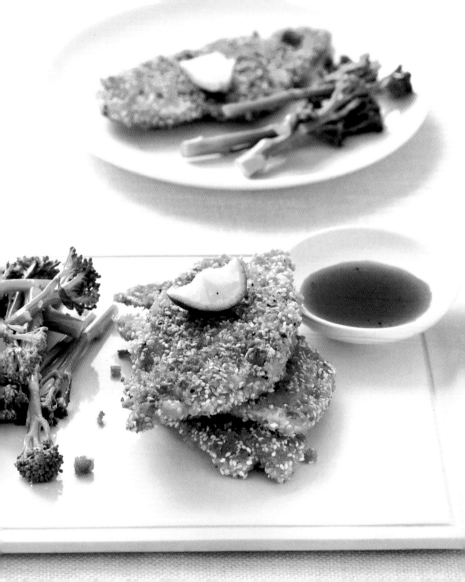

Wasabi is a Japanese root vegetable that is finely grated to make a hot paste a little like horseradish. You could use English mustard or freshly grated horseradish instead, if you prefer.

Soy tuna with wasabi mash

3 tbsp soy sauce
1 tbsp rice wine vinegar
1 tbsp caster sugar
2 tuna steaks, about 140g/5oz each
500g/1lb 2oz potatoes,
peeled and halved
100ml/3½fl oz semi-skimmed milk
2 tsp wasabi paste
1 spring onion, finely sliced
frozen broad beans or soya beans,
to serve

Takes 25 minutes, plus marinating
Serves 2

1 Mix together the soy sauce, vinegar and sugar. Pour over the tuna and marinate for at least 20 minutes or up to 2 hours in the fridge. Put the potatoes in a pan of lightly salted boiling water, then cook for 10–15 minutes until soft. Drain well. Heat the milk in the pan and mix in the wasabi, return the potatoes to the pan, then mash until smooth. Stir through the spring onion and keep warm.
2 Heat a non-stick griddle pan until smoking hot. Remove the tuna from the marinade. Cook on the griddle for 2–3 minutes on each side until seared on the outside but still pink inside. Cook the broad or soya beans according to the packet instructions, then serve alongside the tuna and mash.

• Per serving 439 kcalories, protein 43g, carbohydrate 51g, fat 9g, saturated fat 2g, fibre 3g, sugar 7g, salt 1.38g

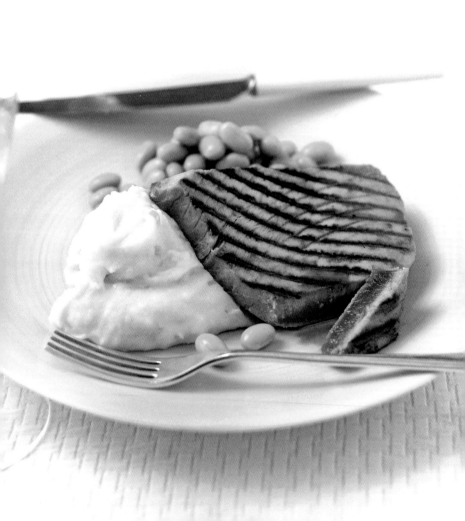

Softening the aubergine in the microwave cuts down the amount of oil that's usually used when frying them for this dish. Remember to prick holes in the aubergine with a fork so that it doesn't explode!

Must-make moussaka

500g pack lean minced beef
1 large aubergine
150g pot 0% fat Greek yogurt
1 egg, beaten
3 tbsp finely grated Parmesan
400g can chopped tomatoes with garlic and herbs
4 tbsp sun-dried tomato purée
400g/14oz leftover boiled potatoes or 350g/12oz uncooked weight, boiled

Takes 30 minutes • Serves 4

1 Preheat the grill to high. Brown the beef in a deep ovenproof frying pan over a high heat for 5 minutes.

2 Meanwhile, prick the aubergine with a fork, then microwave on High for 3–5 minutes until soft. Mix the yogurt, egg and Parmesan together, then add a little seasoning. Set aside.

3 Stir the tomatoes, purée and potatoes in with the beef with some seasoning, and heat through. Smooth the surface of the beef mixture with the back of a spoon, then slice the cooked aubergine and arrange on top. Pour the yogurt mixture over the aubergines, smooth out evenly, then grill until the topping has set and turned golden.

• Per serving 342 kcalories, protein 41g, carbohydrate 25g, fat 9g, saturated fat 4g, fibre 4g, sugar 6g, salt 0.97g

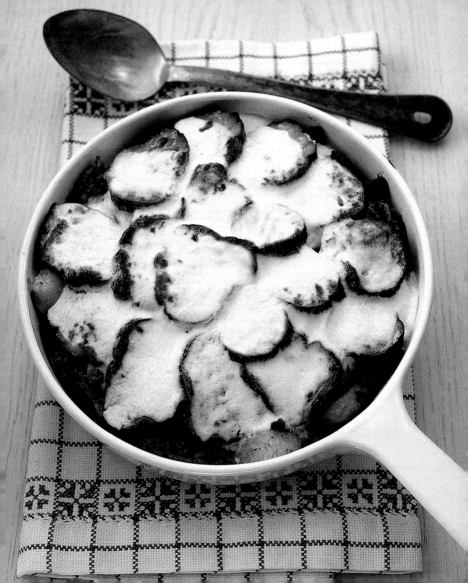

This crispy crumb-topped chicken recipe is a low-fat dish that all the family will enjoy, or make it for an easy supper for friends.

Tomato and crispy-crumb chicken

4 skinless chicken breasts
2 thick slices wholemeal bread
2 tsp dried mixed herbs
400g can chopped tomatoes
1 garlic clove, crushed
1 tsp balsamic vinegar
2 tsp tomato purée
350g/12oz frozen green beans
a handful of flatleaf parsley, chopped, to garnish

Takes 45 minutes • Serves 4

1 Preheat the oven to 190°C/170°C fan/ gas 5. Split the chicken breasts almost in half and open them out like a book. Put in a non-stick roasting tin.
2 Whiz the bread into crumbs in a food processor, then mix with the herbs. Mix the tomatoes with the garlic, vinegar and tomato purée.
3 Spread the tomato sauce over the chicken, sprinkle with the crumbs, then bake for 20–25 minutes until the chicken is tender.
4 While the chicken is cooking, boil the frozen beans for 3–5 minutes until just tender. Serve the chicken, sprinkled with parsley, on a bed of beans.

• Per serving 238 kcalories, protein 39g, carbohydrate 16g, fat 3g, saturated fat 1g, fibre 4g, sugar 5g, salt 0.66g

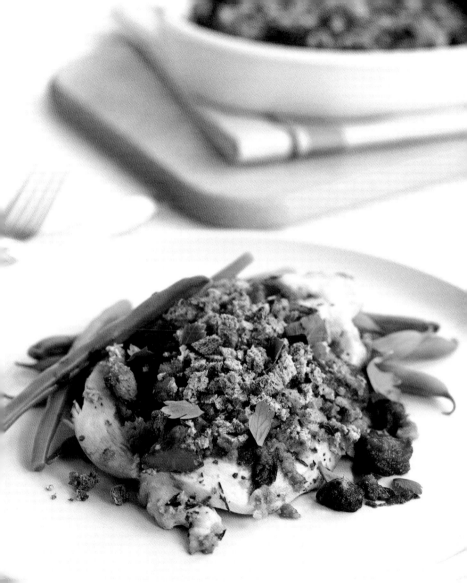

Turn chilli into something special by serving it in roasted butternut-squash halves. The chilli combines beautifully with the sweet squash flesh.

Butternut squash with spicy chilli

2 small butternut squash, halved lengthways and seeds scraped out
1 tbsp olive oil
1 red onion, chopped
2 red chillies, seeded and finely chopped
2 tsp ground cumin
250g/9oz lean minced beef
2 tbsp tomato purée
410g can kidney beans, drained and rinsed
½ × 20g bunch coriander, leaves chopped
50g/2oz baby leaf spinach

Takes 55 minutes • Serves 4

1 Preheat the oven to 200°C/180°C fan/gas 6. Rub the squash halves with a little oil, then roast them on a baking sheet for 45 minutes until soft.
2 Meanwhile, heat the remaining oil in a large frying pan, then fry the onion for a few minutes until soft. Stir in the chillies and cumin, fry for 1 minute more, then add the mince, browning for 3–4 minutes. Stir in the purée and beans with a splash of water and season. Warm through and keep warm.
3 Scoop out a little of the soft squash flesh to make a hollow, then stir this into the chilli with half the coriander. Fill the cavity of each squash with a quarter of the mix, then scatter with the remaining coriander. Dress the spinach with a drop more olive oil, season and serve alongside the squash.

• Per serving 318 kcalories, protein 23g, carbohydrate 37g, fat 10g, saturated fat 3g, fibre 9g, sugar 16g, salt 0.92g

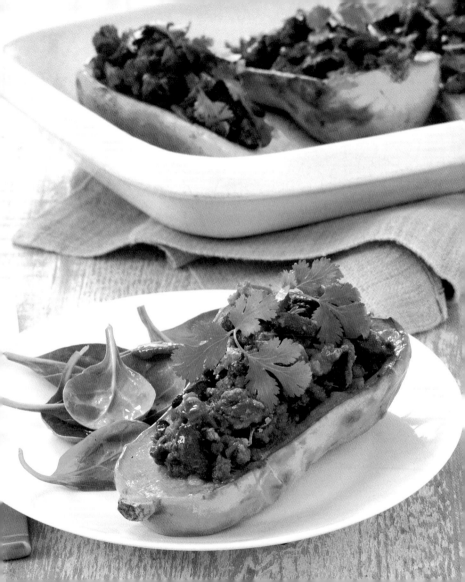

This great-tasting dish is full of fresh, warm flavours. It's a perfect recipe for a spicy casual supper with friends.

Easy Indian chicken with coleslaw

a large handful of coriander, stems finely chopped, leaves separated
2 tsp ground cumin
zest and juice of 2 limes
2 tbsp vegetable oil
4 skinless chicken quarters
1 tbsp ground turmeric
½ small head purple cabbage, shredded
2 carrots, finely shredded
naan bread or rice, to serve (optional)

Takes 1 hour, plus marinating
Serves 4

1 Mix the coriander stems with the cumin, lime zest and juice, and oil. Make three slashes in each chicken quarter, then sprinkle over the turmeric and half the lime mixture. Season well, then leave to marinate for 10 minutes or up to 24 hours in the fridge.
2 Preheat the oven to 200°C/180°C fan/ gas 6 a little while before you are ready to cook the chicken. Roast on a baking sheet for 50 minutes until the chicken is golden and cooked through.
3 Tip the cabbage and carrots into a bowl, then pour over the remaining lime dressing. Add the coriander leaves and toss. Serve alongside the chicken with some warm naan bread or rice, if you like.

• Per serving 147 kcalories, protein 11g, carbohydrate 9g, fat 8g, saturated fat 1g, fibre 2g, sugar 5g, salt 0.16g

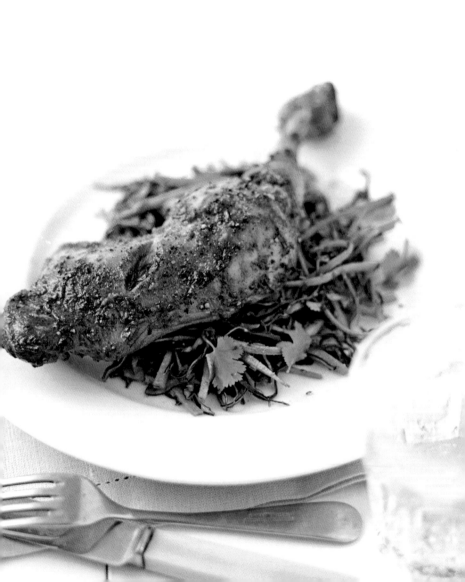

Trout is a good source of heart-healthy omega-3s.
Here the fish is cooked in a paper parcel with vegetables
so it both looks and tastes great.

Trout en papillote

2 large carrots, cut into batons
3 celery sticks, cut into batons
1 tbsp olive oil
½ tsp sugar
6 tbsp white wine
4 trout fillets, about 175g/6oz each
a few basil leaves, to scatter
juice of 1 lemon

Takes 45 minutes • Serves 4

1 Preheat the oven to 190°C/170°C fan/ gas 5. Put the carrots and celery in a pan with the oil, sugar, wine, salt and pepper. Bring to the boil, tightly cover, then cook for 10 minutes until the vegetables are tender. Leave to cool.

2 Cut four large sheets of baking parchment, about 35cm square. Divide the vegetables among them and top each with a trout fillet. Scatter a few basil leaves and a little lemon juice over each, then season the fish with a little salt and pepper. Fold the paper in half and double fold all round to seal in the fish, a bit like a pasty.

3 Put the parcels on two baking sheets and bake for 15–20 minutes (depending on the thickness of the fish). Serve in their paper with some steamed new potatoes.

• Per serving 262 kcalories, protein 35g, carbohydrate 8g, fat 10g, saturated fat 2g, fibre 2g, sugar 7g, salt 0.37g

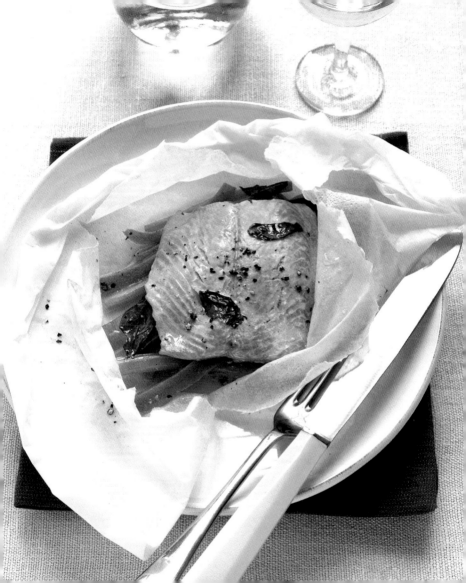

This tomato-based spicy fish stew is so simple to cook yet looks really impressive for a special dinner for two.

Summer seafood simmer

8 large raw prawns
1 tbsp olive oil
1 small onion, finely chopped
2 garlic cloves, crushed
1 tsp hot smoked paprika
200ml/7fl oz dry white wine
400g can chopped tomatoes
1 roasted red pepper, from
a jar, sliced
200g/8oz skinless boneless white
fish fillets, cut into chunks
a handful of chopped parsley
crusty bread, to serve

Takes 40 minutes • Serves 2

1 Peel the prawns and de-vein them by simply scoring down the back and removing the black vein. Set aside.
2 Heat the olive oil in a heavy-based pan, then add the onion. Cook gently for 3–4 minutes until softened, then add the garlic and paprika. Cook for a further minute, then pour in the wine. Allow to bubble for a minute or so, then tip in the tomatoes. Season, then leave to simmer for 20 minutes.
3 Stir the red pepper, fish and prawns into the stew. Simmer gently for 4–5 minutes, or until the fish and prawns are cooked through. Stir in the chopped parsley, then serve with crusty bread.

• Per serving 353 kcalories, protein 38g, carbohydrate 16g, fat 12g, saturated fat 2g, fibre 4g, sugar 13g, salt 1.74g

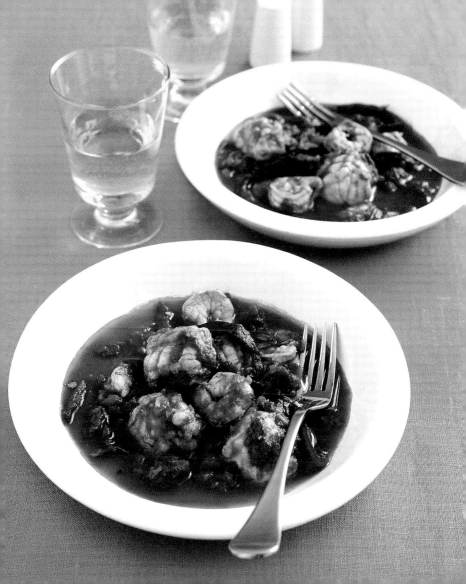

These tasty home-made burgers use extra-lean beef mince lightened with couscous and flavoured with herbs and chilli. Serve on a slice of French bread.

Leanburgers with rocket and peppers

50g/2oz couscous
500g/1lb 2oz extra lean minced beef
1 small onion, finely chopped
2 tsp mixed dried herbs
3 tbsp snipped chives
¼ tsp hot chilli powder
6 slices French bread
6 tsp Dijon mustard
175g/6oz roasted red peppers from a jar, cut into large pieces (choose ones in brine, or rinse them if they're packed in oil)
a couple of handfuls of rocket leaves

Takes 25–35 minutes • Serves 6

1 Tip the couscous into a medium bowl, pour over 75ml/3fl oz boiling water and leave it for a few minutes to swell and absorb all the water.

2 Add the mince, onion, dried herbs, chives and chilli powder, then grind in plenty of salt and pepper. Mix thoroughly then shape into six oval burgers that are slightly larger than the bread slices. Cover with foil and chill until ready to cook.

3 Heat the grill or barbecue, then cook the burgers for 5–6 minutes on each side, or more if you like them well cooked.

4 Grill or lightly toast the slices of bread and spread with the mustard. Top with the peppers, rocket and a burger, and serve.

• Per serving 260 kcalories, protein 23g, carbohydrate 30g, fat 6g, saturated fat 2g, fibre 2g, sugar none, salt 1.1g

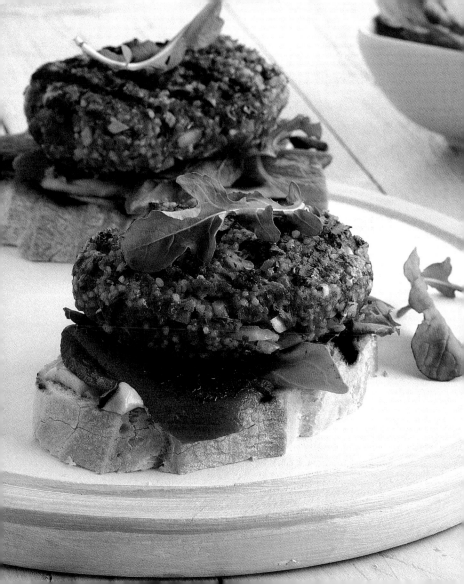

Snapper or sea bass would also work well in this recipe,
though as they can be quite expensive, use trout, which works
a treat with gentle aromatic flavours.

Baked fish with Thai spices

4 trout fillets, about 200g/8oz each
1 lemongrass stalk, finely chopped
small knob of ginger, peeled
and finely chopped
1 red chilli, seeded and
finely chopped
1 garlic clove, finely chopped
1 tbsp fish sauce
juice of 2 limes
1 tsp golden caster sugar
a handful of coriander, roughly
chopped

Takes 20 minutes • Serves 4

1 Preheat the oven to 200°C/180°C fan/
gas 6. Tear off two large sheets of foil and
put one fillet, skin-side down, in the centre of
each sheet. Make a sauce by mixing together
the remaining ingredients. Spoon half of
this mixture over the fillets, setting aside the
remainder.
2 Put the other two fish fillets on top of each
fillet to make a sandwich, skin-side up, then
tightly seal the foil to create two packages.
Bake in the oven for 12–15 minutes. Bring
the packages to the table to open and serve
with the rest of the sauce.

• Per serving 236 kcalories, protein 40g, carbohydrate
2g, fat 8g, saturated fat 2g, fibre none, sugar 1g,
salt 1.02g

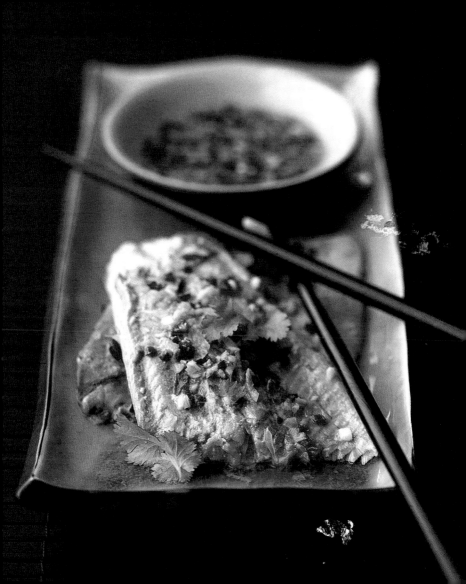

Beef skirt has an excellent flavour and is best served rare to medium rare or it becomes tough. Skirt can also be used for braising.

Garlic beef

1 tbsp black peppercorns
6 garlic cloves
4 tbsp red wine vinegar
600g/1lb 5oz piece well-trimmed beef skirt
chips and mustard, to serve (optional)

Takes 25 minutes, plus marinating
Serves 4

1 In a pestle and mortar, crush the peppercorns and garlic with a pinch of salt until you have a smooth-ish paste, then stir in the vinegar. Sit the beef in a non-metallic dish, then rub all over with the paste. Leave in the fridge for a few hours, but no longer.
2 To cook, put a griddle pan over a very high heat. Rub the marinade off the meat, then season with a little more salt. Cook the meat until charred on each side – about 5 minutes per side for rare, longer if you prefer it medium or well done. If the cut is very thick, you may want to roast it in a hot oven for 5 minutes after searing.
3 Lift on to a chopping board, then rest for 5 minutes before carving into slices and serving with chips, if you like.

• Per serving 205 kcalories, protein 34g, carbohydrate 3g, fat 6g, saturated fat 2g, fibre none, sugar none, salt 0.24g

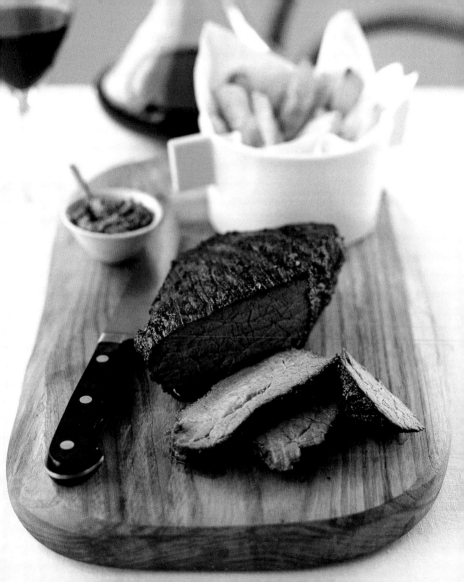

Asian cooking can be light, healthy and so quick that you'll think twice before ever ordering a take-away again. Sprinkle with sesame seeds if you have some in your storecupboard.

Chicken stir-fry

1 egg white
1 tbsp cornflour, plus 1 tsp extra
4 skinless chicken breasts, sliced
350g/12oz Thai fragrant rice
1 tbsp vegetable oil
1 red pepper, seeded and cut into chunks
1 tbsp finely chopped ginger
1 shallot, thinly sliced
1 garlic clove, thinly sliced
1 red chilli, seeded and sliced (optional)
1 tbsp fish sauce
juice of 1 lime
a handful of basil leaves

Takes 35 minutes, plus marinating
Serves 4

1 Beat together the egg white and the 1 tablespoon of cornflour. Mix in the chicken and marinate for 15–30 minutes.
2 Rinse and drain the rice, tip into a pan and pour over 600ml/1 pint of water and a pinch of salt. Bring to the boil, then cook for 10 minutes or so until the water has almost boiled away. Cover, turn the heat down low and cook for 10 minutes more.
3 Remove the chicken from the marinade and pat dry. Heat the oil in a wok and cook the chicken for 7–10 minutes, tossing until cooked. Set aside. Add the pepper and cook for 1 minute, then add the ginger, shallot, garlic and chilli, if using, for 1–2 minutes more.
4 Combine the fish sauce, lime juice, 50ml/2fl oz water and the 1 teaspoon of cornflour. Tip into the wok with the chicken. Cook for 1 minute, stir through the basil, then serve with the rice.

• Per serving 501 kcalories, protein 42g, carbohydrate 76g, fat 5g, saturated fat 1g, fibre 2g, sugar 3g, salt 1.02g

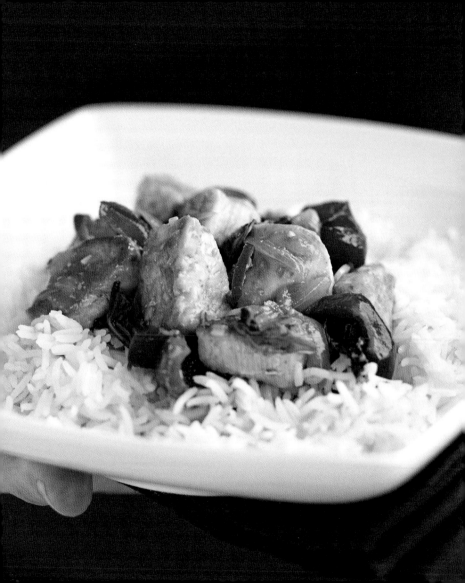

A new way to serve steak – marinated in a soy-and-honey mix then griddled and served with a crunchy salad.

Teriyaki steak with fennel slaw

2 tbsp reduced-salt soy sauce
1 tbsp red wine vinegar
1 tsp clear honey
4 sirloin or rump steaks, trimmed of all visible fat, about 125g/4½oz each

FOR THE FENNEL SLAW
1 large carrot, coarsely grated
1 fennel bulb, halved and thinly sliced
1 red onion, halved and thinly sliced
a handful of coriander leaves
juice of 1 lime

Takes 20 minutes, plus marinating
Serves 4

1 Mix the soy, vinegar and honey, add the steaks, then marinate for 10–15 minutes.
2 Toss together the carrot, fennel, onion and coriander, then chill until ready to serve.
3 Remove the steaks from the marinade, reserving the liquid on one side. Cook the steaks in a griddle pan for a few minutes on each side, depending on the thickness and how well done you like them. Set the meat aside to rest on a plate, then add the remaining marinade to the pan. Bubble the marinade until it reduces a little to make a sticky sauce.
4 Dress the slaw with the lime juice, then pile on to plates and serve with the steaks. Spoon the sauce over the meat.

• Per serving 188 kcalories, protein 29g, carbohydrate 7g, fat 5g, saturated fat 2g, fibre 2g, sugar 6g, salt 1.05g

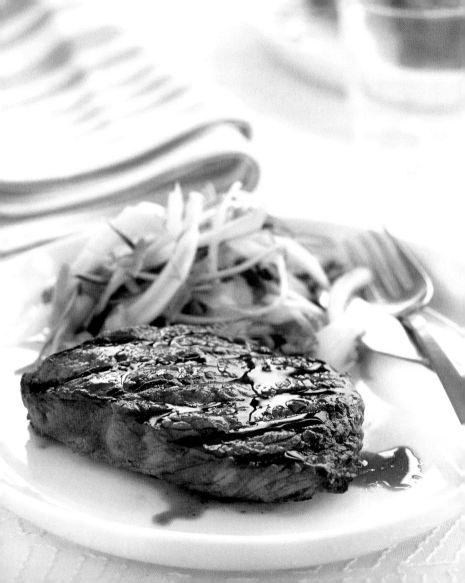

A great Saturday-night supper – fresh, light and tangy fish
served with crunchy chips.

Healthy fish and chips
with tartare sauce

450g/1lb potatoes, peeled and
cut into chips
1 tbsp olive oil, plus a little
extra for brushing
2 white fish fillets, about
140g/5oz each
grated zest and juice of 1 lemon
a small handful of parsley leaves,
chopped
1 tbsp capers, chopped
2 heaped tbsp 0% fat Greek yogurt

Takes 40–45 minutes • Serves 2

1 Preheat the oven to 200°C/180°C fan/
gas 6. Toss the prepared chips in the oil.
Spread over a baking sheet in an even layer
and bake for 40 minutes until browned and
crisp.
2 Put the fish in a shallow dish, brush lightly
with oil, salt and pepper. Sprinkle with half the
lemon juice, bake for 12–15 minutes. After
10 minutes, sprinkle over the lemon zest and
a little of the parsley to finish cooking.
3 Meanwhile, mix the capers, yogurt,
remaining parsley and lemon juice together,
set aside, and season to taste.
4 To serve, divide the chips between plates,
lift the fish on to the plates and serve with a
little side dish of the tartare sauce.

• Per serving 373 kcalories, protein 35g, carbohydrate
41g, fat 9g, saturated fat 1g, fibre 3g, added sugar
none, salt 0.96g

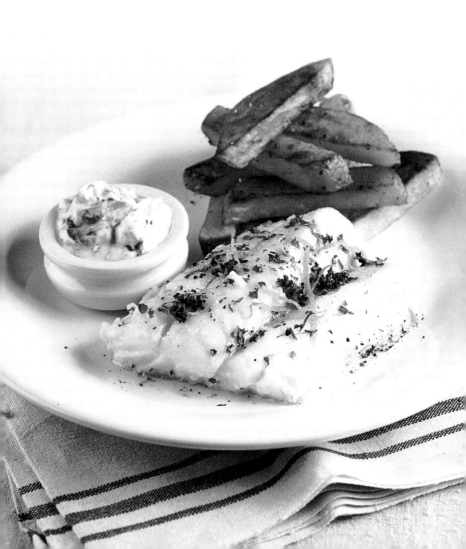

This is a one-pot dish, as everything is cooked in a Chinese bamboo steamer. If you don't have a steamer, cook it in a foil parcel in a medium oven for 30 minutes.

Steamed bass with pak choi

small knob of ginger,
peeled and sliced
2 garlic cloves, finely sliced
3 spring onions, finely sliced
2 tbsp soy sauce
1 tbsp sesame oil
splash of sherry (optional)
2 sea bass fillets, about
140g/5oz each
2 pak choi heads, quartered

Takes 15 minutes • Serves 2

1 In a small bowl, combine all of the ingredients, except the fish and the pak choi, to make a soy mix. Line one tier of a two-tiered bamboo steamer loosely with foil. Lay the fish, skin-side up, on the foil and spoon over the soy mix. Put the fish over a pan of simmering water and throw the pak choi into the second tier then cover it with a lid. Alternatively, add the pak choi to the fish layer after 2 minutes of cooking – the closer the tier is to the steam, the hotter it is.
2 Leave everything to steam for 6–8 minutes until the pak choi has wilted and the fish is cooked. Divide the greens between two plates, then carefully lift out the fish. Lift the foil up and drizzle the tasty juices back over the fish.

• Per serving 217 kcalories, protein 30g, carbohydrate 5g, fat 9g, saturated fat 1g, fibre none, sugar 2g, salt 4.58g

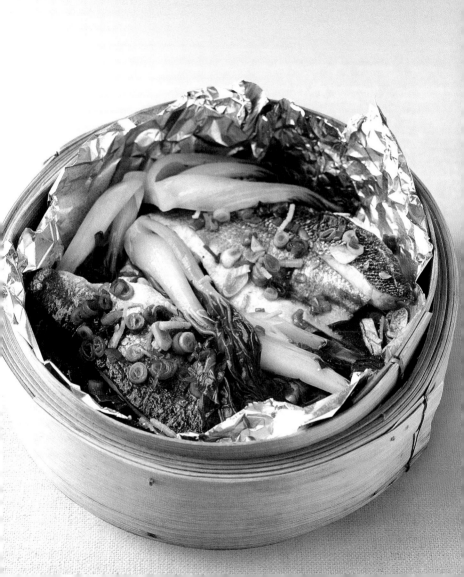

Rice pudding can be made in the microwave in under 20 minutes. For a change, stir in a handful of blueberries instead of the banana.

Banana rice pudding with cinnamon sugar

1 tbsp custard powder
400ml/14fl oz skimmed milk
2 tbsp demerara sugar
1 large banana, thinly sliced
85g/3oz pudding rice
¼ tsp ground cinnamon

Takes 17 minutes • Serves 2

1 Put the custard powder into a large, deep microwaveable dish with a lid, then mix to a paste with a dribble of the milk. Stir in the rest of the milk gradually so you have no custardy lumps, then add 1 tablespoon of the sugar and half the banana. Cover tightly with the lid and microwave for 3 minutes on High. Stir in the rice, cover again, then microwave on High for 6 minutes, stirring halfway through.
2 Carefully stir in the remaining banana – take care as the rice will be very hot. Cover and microwave for 4 minutes more, stirring at 1-minute intervals to check if the rice is cooked. Cooking times will vary a little, depending on your microwave.
3 Meanwhile, mix the remaining sugar and cinnamon together. Spoon the creamy banana rice into two bowls and serve sprinkled with the crunchy cinnamon sugar.

• Per serving 347 kcalories, protein 11g, carbohydrate 78g, fat 1g, saturated fat none, fibre 1g, sugar 37g, salt 0.29g

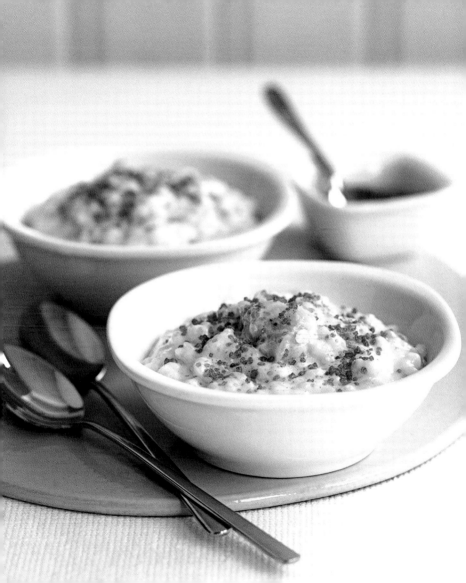

Intensely fruity, lightly spiced apricots are the perfect foil
for creamy Greek yogurt. Try serving these light low-fat puddings
with delicate brandy snaps.

Apricot yogurt fool

600g/1lb 5oz ripe apricots, halved
and stoned
juice of 1 large orange
50g/2oz caster sugar
2 cinnamon sticks, broken
500g pot Greek yogurt
zest of 1 lemon

Takes 20 minutes, plus cooling
Serves 4

1 Put the apricots, orange juice, sugar
and cinnamon sticks in a pan, cover and
cook gently for about 15 minutes, until the
apricots are very soft. Remove the cinnamon
sticks and set aside the fruit to cool.
2 Spoon the yogurt into a bowl and stir in
the lemon zest. Fold in most of the cooled
apricots, divide among into four serving
glasses and spoon over the remaining fruit
and any juices.

• Per serving 246 kcalories, protein 9g, carbohydrate
28g, fat 11g, saturated fat 7g, fibre 3g, added sugar
13g, salt 0.24g

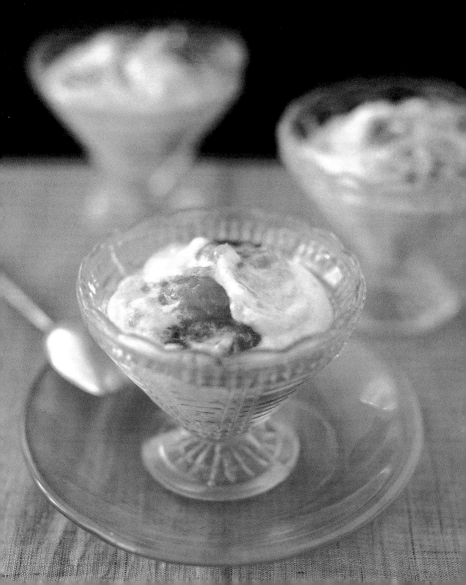

Top these little puds with whatever fruit you've got at home.
For a delicious banoffee version, slice bananas and toss with
a squeeze of fresh lemon juice and a spoonful of caramel sauce.

Strawberry cheesecakes

85g/3oz low-fat biscuits
200g tub extra-light soft cheese
200g pot 0% fat Greek yogurt
4 tbsp caster sugar
a few drops vanilla extract
2 tbsp good-quality strawberry jam
100g/4oz strawberries, hulled
and sliced

Takes 10 minutes • Serves 4

1 Put the biscuits in a plastic bag and
bash with a rolling pin until you have chunky
crumbs. Divide among four glasses or
small bowls.
2 Beat the soft cheese, yogurt, sugar and
vanilla together until smooth, then spoon over
the crumbs, and chill until ready to serve.
3 Stir the jam in a bowl until loose, then
gently stir in the strawberries. Divide the
strawberries among the cheesecakes
and serve.

• Per serving 263 kcalories, protein 12g, carbohydrate
43g, fat 6g, saturated fat 3g, fibre 1g, sugar 31g,
salt 0.93g

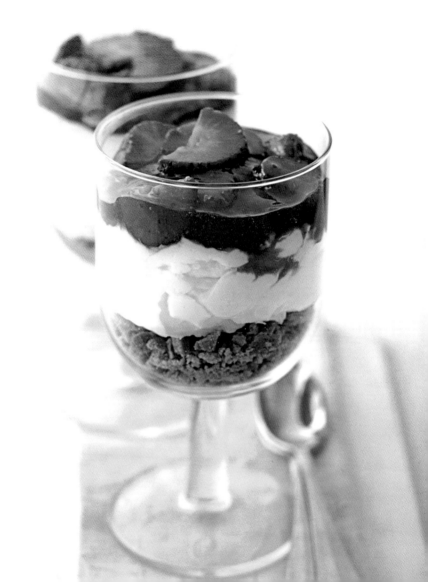

The cooking time will vary depending on the ripeness of the fruit, so keep an eye on the pan. Peaches would also work well in this recipe.

Poached apricots with rosewater

50g/2oz golden caster sugar
400g/14oz ripe apricots, halved
and stoned
a few drops rosewater
Greek yogurt and a handful of
pistachios, roughly chopped,
to decorate

Takes 20 minutes, plus cooling
Serves 2

1 Put the sugar into a medium pan with 150ml/¼ pint water. Heat gently until the sugar dissolves, then add the apricots and simmer for 15 minutes until soft.
2 Take off the heat, splash in the rosewater and leave to cool. Spoon into two glasses and serve topped with a few dollops of the yogurt and a scattering of nuts.

• Per serving 161 kcalories, protein 2g, carbohydrate 41g, fat none, saturated fat none, fibre 3g, sugar 41g, salt 0.01g

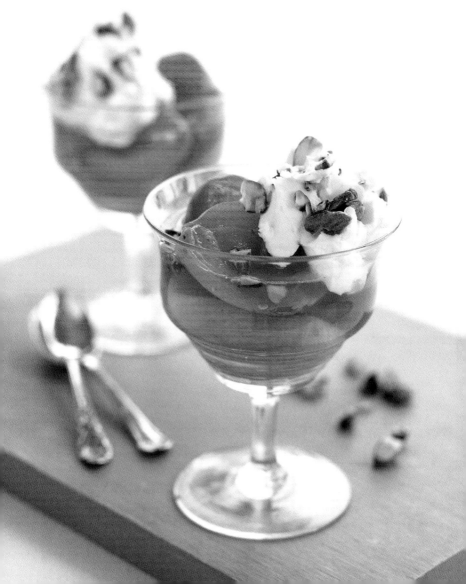

Make this wonderfully healthy dish and eat it at any time of day as a great pick-me-up, or add a good dollop of mascarpone to transform it into a quick pudding.

Warm winter fruit with chestnuts

100g/4oz light muscovado sugar
3 wide strips orange zest
1 vanilla pod, split lengthways
140g/5oz cooked chestnuts
100g/4oz dried cherries
100g/4oz dried apricots
mascarpone, to serve (optional)

Takes 25 minutes • Serves 6

1 Put the sugar, orange zest and vanilla in a pan with 200ml/7fl oz water. Bring to the boil, stirring to dissolve the sugar, then add the chestnuts and dried fruits. Simmer, uncovered, for 10 minutes until the syrup is slightly thickened.

2 Leave to cool, then serve with spoonfuls of mascarpone, if you like.

• Per serving 185 kcalories, protein 2g, carbohydrate 46g, fat 1g, saturated fat none, fibre 3g, sugar 38g, salt 0.05g

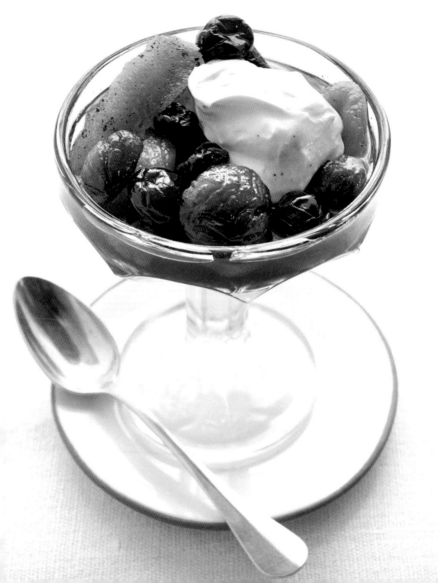

Ginger is a delicious partner to rhubarb, and this put-together dessert
takes just 5 minutes to layer into pretty serving glasses.

Crunchy spiced rhubarb trifles

540g can rhubarb
a pinch of ground ginger
500g tub fresh custard
6 ginger nut biscuits, roughly
crushed

Takes 5 minutes • Serves 4

1 Mix the rhubarb and ginger together, and divide among four serving glasses.
2 Spoon the custard on top (you will have some left over) and finish with a sprinkling of crushed biscuit.

• Per serving 254 kcalories, protein 5g, carbohydrate 42g, fat 10g, saturated fat 5g, fibre 1g, sugar 18g, salt 0.3g

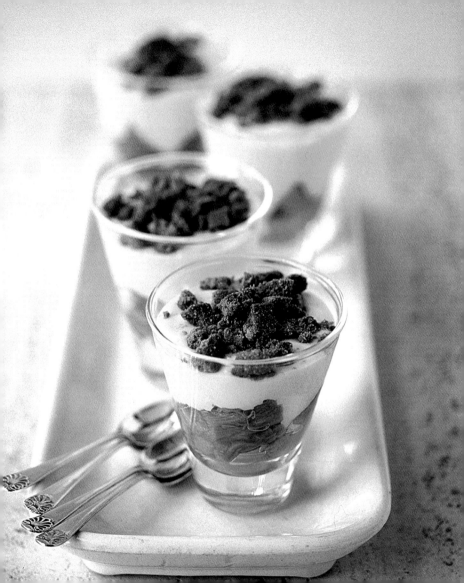

Serve warm for pudding or cool the pears in the fridge overnight, then enjoy with muesli or crunchy oat cereal and yogurt for breakfast.

Maple pears with pecans and cranberries

4 ripe pears
a handful of dried cranberries
2 tbsp maple syrup, plus extra to drizzle (optional)
50g/2oz pecan nuts, roughly chopped
Greek yogurt, to serve

Takes 10 minutes • Serves 4

1 Peel and halve the pears, and scoop out the core with a teaspoon. Lay the halves in a shallow microwaveable dish, cut-side down, along with the cranberries. Pour the 2 tablespoons of maple syrup over and cover with cling film. Microwave on High for 3 minutes until softened, stirring halfway through. Uncover and leave to cool for a few minutes. Stir the pecan nuts through the syrup.
2 Spoon into serving dishes, drizzle with extra maple syrup, if you like, and serve with Greek yogurt.

• Per serving 208 kcalories, protein 2g, carbohydrate 32g, fat 9g, saturated fat 1g, fibre 4g, sugar 9g, salt none

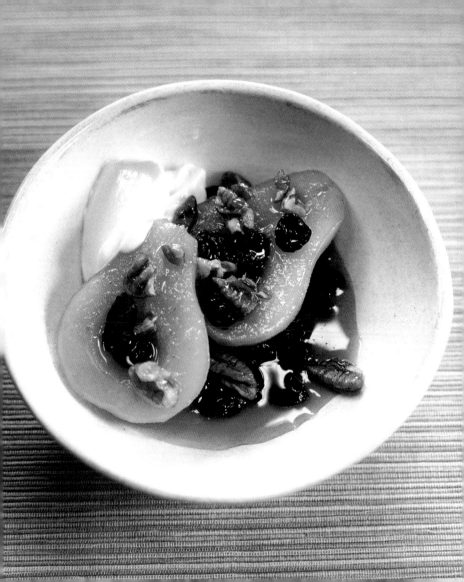

These little French vanilla custard puddings are deliciously creamy and surprisingly low in fat. They will keep in the fridge for up to 2 days.

Oeufs au lait

butter, for greasing
425ml/¾ pint milk
85g/3oz caster sugar
1 sachet vanilla sugar or
1 tsp vanilla extract
2 eggs

Takes 40 minutes, plus chilling
Serves 4

1 Butter four ramekins, about 150ml/¼ pint each. Preheat the oven to 160°C/140°C fan/gas 3. Have a roasting tin ready and put the kettle on.

2 Pour the milk into a pan with the sugar and vanilla. Bring gently to the boil, stirring to dissolve the sugar. Remove from the heat and cool for a few minutes.

3 In a large bowl, beat the eggs until frothy. Slowly whisk in the milk. Set the ramekins in the roasting tin and divide the custard among them. Pour hot water around the ramekins to come halfway up the sides. Bake for 20 minutes until just set, then cool and chill before serving.

• Per serving 181 kcalories, protein 7g, carbohydrate 28g, fat 5g, saturated fat 2g, fibre none, sugar 23g, salt 0.23g

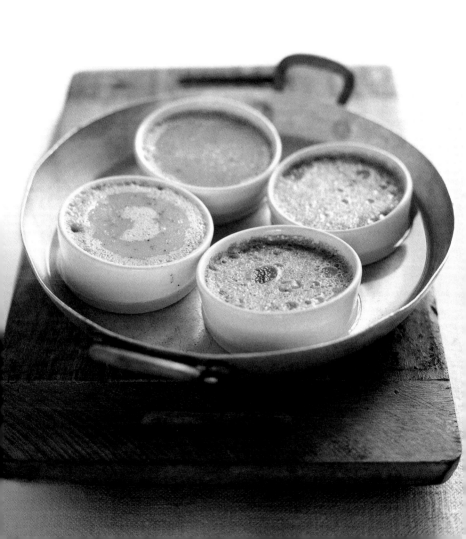

If you have a gluten or wheat intolerance, try these summer puddings made with gluten-free bread. We made the leftover bread (from cutting the circles) into breadcrumbs and froze them for future use.

Summer puddings

250g punnet strawberries, hulled
and halved
125g punnet blueberries
125g punnet blackberries
85g/3oz golden caster sugar
6 thin slices bread from a
gluten-free loaf

Takes 35 minutes, plus chilling
Serves 4

1 Put the fruit into a large pan with the sugar and 3 tablespoons water. Heat on low for 2–3 minutes until the juice runs from the fruit. Remove from the heat.

2 Using biscuit cutters, stamp out four 5.5cm circles from the bread, then use a 7-cm cutter for another four circles. Put the smaller circles into the base of four 175ml/6fl oz pudding basins. Spoon in the fruit, then top with the larger circles. Press down, then spoon over just enough juice to colour the bread red, reserving any remaining juice. Cover with cling film and put a weight (such as a jar of jam) on top. Chill for at least 4 hours.

3 To serve the puddings, uncover and run a knife around the edge. Put a serving plate over each one, then invert and spoon over the reserved juice.

• Per serving 212 kcalories, protein 1g, carbohydrate 52g, fat 1g, saturated fat none, fibre 2g, added sugar 22g, salt 0.53g

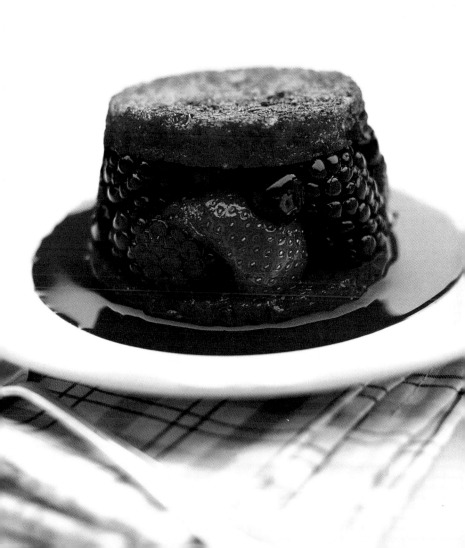

This show-stopper jelly makes a great finale to a meal.
For a grown-up dinner party add 100ml/3½fl oz vodka
to both of the fruit juices.

Cranberry sunrise

10 sheets leaf gelatine
700ml/1¼ pint smooth-style
orange juice, warmed through
700ml/1¼ pint cranberry juice,
warmed through

Takes 10 minutes, plus overnight
setting • Serves 8–10

1 Soak 5 leaf gelatine sheets in cold water
for at least 5 minutes until soft. Drain the
gelatine and squeeze to get rid of any
excess water. Dissolve the soaked gelatine
in 100ml/3½fl oz hot water from the kettle.
Add to the warm orange juice and set aside.
Repeat the process, this time using the warm
cranberry juice.
2 Pour half of the orange juice into a large
jelly mould and chill in the fridge until set
completely – about 4 hours. Cover the
orange jelly with half the cranberry juice and
chill to set. Repeat the process until both
juices are used. Leave to set overnight.

• Per serving 110 kcalories, protein 5g, carbohydrate
24g, fat none, saturated fat none, fibre none, added
sugar 10g, salt 0.1g

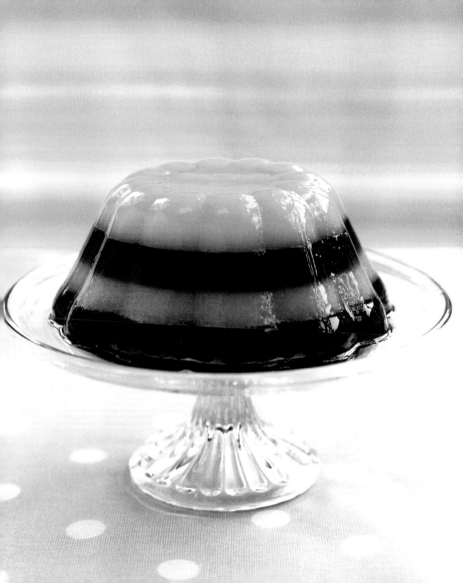

This dessert brings back memories of childhood, as the taste is reminiscent of the milk lollies we used to enjoy so much.

Vanilla jellies with apricot and raspberry compote

4 sheets leaf gelatine
600ml/1 pint milk
50g/2oz caster sugar, plus 2 tbsp for compote
2 tsp vanilla extract or rosewater
500g/1lb 2oz apricots
3 tbsp apple juice
100g/4oz raspberries

Takes 30 minutes, plus chilling
Serves 4

1 Soak the gelatine for 10 minutes in enough cold water to cover the leaves. Bring the milk and the 50g/2oz of sugar slowly to the boil, gently stirring to dissolve the sugar. Remove from the heat and stir in the vanilla extract or rosewater.

2 Remove the gelatine from its soaking water, squeeze out the water, then stir into the milk until it has dissolved. Pour the jellies into four 150ml moulds, cups or ramekins. Cool, then chill until set, about 3 hours.

3 Halve and stone the apricots, then cut each half into four. Put in a pan with the apple juice and the 2 tablespoons of sugar, then bring to a simmer. Gently cook for about 5 minutes until the apricots are tender, but not pulpy. Remove from the heat, stir in the raspberries, then leave to cool.

4 Turn the jellies out on to four plates, then spoon the compote around the edge of each one.

• Per serving 221 kcalories, protein 12g, carbohydrate 40g, fat 3g, saturated fat 2g, fibre 3g, sugar 40g, salt 0.23g

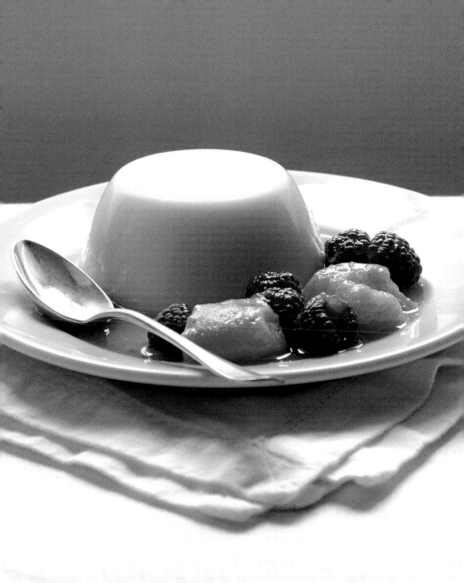

This is a great way of using overripe summer fruits and makes a delicious low-fat pud with its crunchy fruit-loaf topping.

Fruity summer Charlotte

500g/1lb 2oz summer fruit (we used raspberries, blackberries and blueberries)
4 tbsp demerara sugar
7 slices from a small cinnamon and raisin loaf
25g/1oz butter, softened
crème fraîche or fromage frais, to serve

Takes 20 minutes • Serves 4

1 Preheat the oven to 220°C/200°C fan/gas 7. Tumble three-quarters of the berries into a medium baking dish. Whiz the remainder of the berries in a food processor to make a purée, then stir this into the dish along with 2 tablespoons of the sugar.
2 Spread the loaf slices with butter, then cut into triangles. Cover the top of the fruit with the bread slices, then scatter over the rest of the sugar. Cover with foil, bake for 10 minutes, uncover the dish, then bake for 5 minutes more until the fruit is starting to bubble and the bread is toasty. Serve with dollops of crème fraîche or fromage frais.

• Per serving 262 kcalories, protein 6g, carbohydrate 47g, fat 7g, saturated fat 4g, fibre 5g, sugar 33g, salt 0.43g

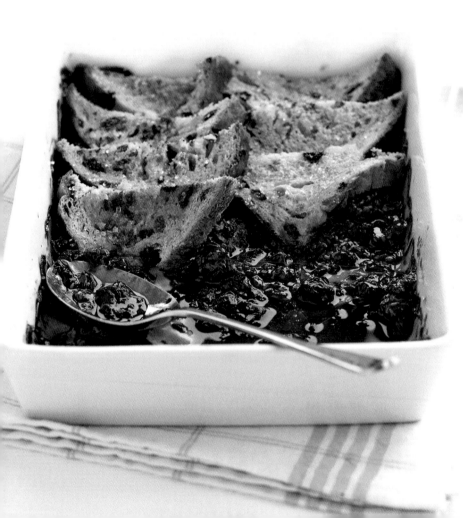

Zabaglione, the sweet Italian 'mousse', is lovely rippled with a few crushed berries for a quick, outstanding dessert. Just delicious!

Blackberry zabaglione

400g/14oz blackberries
140g/5oz golden caster sugar
6 egg yolks
1 vanilla pod
3 tbsp Marsala or sweet wine

Takes 15 minutes • Serves 6

1 In a bowl, lightly crush the berries with 25g/1oz of the sugar. Add a spoonful to the bottom of six small glasses, then set the rest of the berry mixture aside.

2 Bring some water to a gentle simmer in a medium-sized pan and tip the egg yolks into a large heatproof bowl. Halve and scrape the seeds from the vanilla pod into the egg yolks and add the remaining sugar. Using an electric whisk, beat until light and airy. Splash in the Marsala, put the bowl over the pan of simmering water, then whisk your heart out for 10–12 minutes until the egg yolks are thick and foamy and the whisk leaves a defined trail.

3 Drain off some of the juice, then ripple the remaining berries through the mousse and spoon into the glasses.

• Per serving 205 kcalories, protein 5g, carbohydrate 32g, fat 7g, saturated fat 2g, fibre 3g, sugar 32g, salt 0.04g

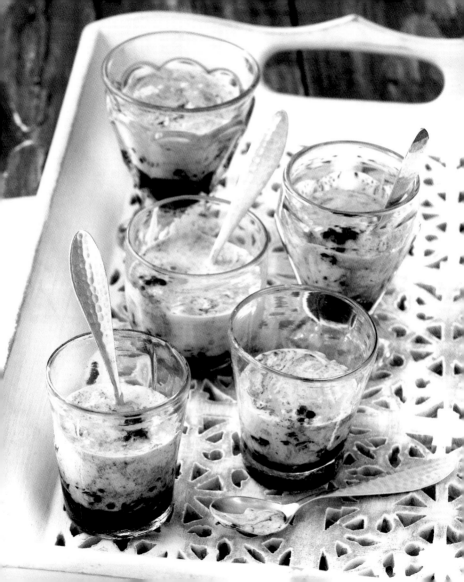

The fromage frais adds a creamy flavour to this pud. For extra crunch, stir through 1 tablespoon each of toasted sesame seeds, pine nuts and pumpkin seeds at the end of cooking.

Apricot and orange rice pudding

200g/8oz pudding rice
600ml/1 pint skimmed milk
a big pinch of ground nutmeg
1 tbsp clear honey, plus
extra to drizzle
140g/5oz ready-to-eat dried apricots,
roughly chopped
zest and juice of 1 orange
4 tbsp reduced-fat fromage frais
a handful of toasted sliced almonds,
to sprinkle

Takes 20 minutes • Serves 4

1 Put the rice, milk and nutmeg into a large microwaveable bowl. Cover with cling film, pierce it, then cook on High for 5 minutes. Stir and leave to stand for 1 minute, then return the bowl to the microwave for a further 5–6 minutes or until the rice is cooked and all the milk absorbed. Remove from the microwave and stand for a further 2 minutes.
2 Put the honey, apricots and orange juice into another microwaveable bowl, and cook on High for 1 minute until the apricots have plumped up. Stir the syrupy apricots, fromage frais and a pinch of the orange zest into the rice.
3 Serve straight away in bowls, topped with a sprinkling of almonds, the remaining orange zest and a drizzle of honey to taste.

• Per serving 325 kcalories, protein 13g, carbohydrate 62g, fat 4g, saturated fat 0.4g, fibre 3g, sugar 24g, salt 0.2g

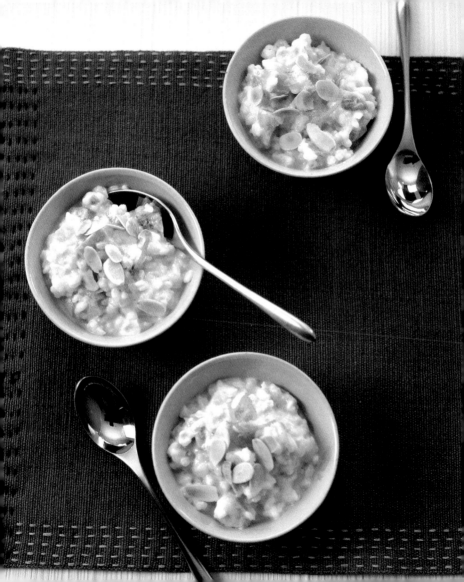

Use any kind of canned fruit in this comfort-food pud.
We used a mixture of cherries and apricot halves.

Sweet and fruity Yorkshire

2 × 400g cans fruit in juice, drained
85g/3oz plain flour
50g/2oz caster sugar
3 eggs, beaten
300ml/½ pint milk
icing sugar, to dust (optional)

Takes 30 minutes • Serves 4

1 Preheat the oven to 220°C/200°C fan/gas 7. Spread the fruit out in a medium baking dish. Combine the flour and caster sugar in a bowl, make a well in the centre, and stir in the eggs until smooth. Gradually stir in the milk until you have a smooth batter, the consistency of pouring cream.

2 Pour the batter over the fruit and bake for 20–25 minutes until golden and set. Dust with icing sugar, if you like, and serve hot or warm.

• Per serving 363 kcalories, protein 11g, carbohydrate 69g, fat 7g, saturated fat 2g, fibre 2g, sugar 53g, salt 0.26g

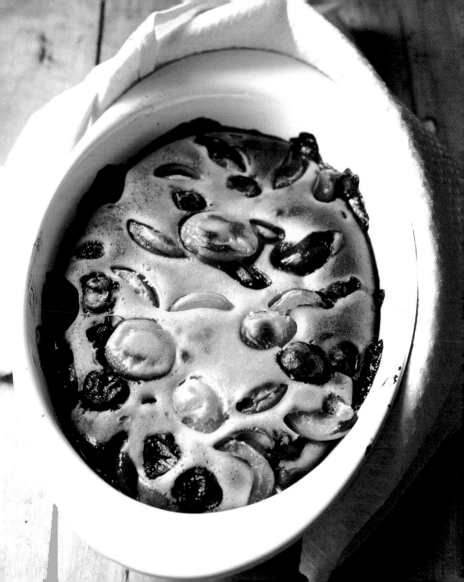

To stop the apples going brown, sprinkle them with a squeeze of lemon juice while you assemble the rest of this simple tart.

No-roll mincemeat and apple tart

25g/1oz golden caster sugar
a generous pinch of ground cinnamon, nutmeg or mixed spice
225g ready-rolled shortcrust pastry, cut into a circle
410g jar mincemeat
2 eating apples, peeled, cored and sliced
custard or ice cream, to serve

Takes 25 minutes • Serves 8

1 Preheat the oven to 220°C/200°C fan/ gas 7. Mix the sugar and spice together in a small bowl. Unroll the pastry on to a flat baking sheet. Spoon the mincemeat in a rough circle over the middle of the pastry, scatter over the apple, then sprinkle with the spiced sugar.
2 Bring the pastry up around the edge of the filling, pressing the folds together with your fingers so that the sides stand up on their own. Bake for 20 minutes until the pastry is golden and the apples have softened. Serve hot or warm with custard or ice cream.

• Per serving 293 kcalories, protein 2g, carbohydrate 52g, fat 10g, saturated fat 4g, fibre 2g, sugar 39g, salt 0.31g

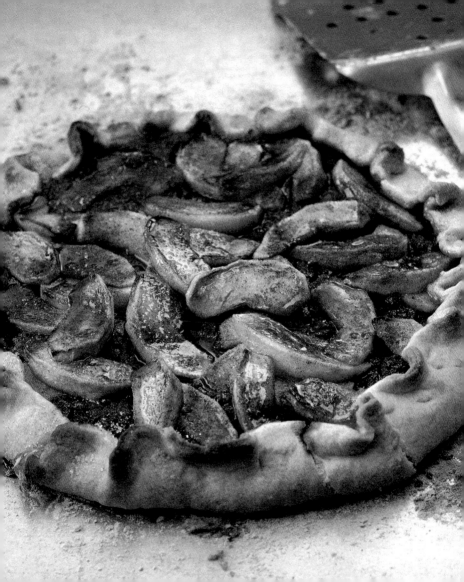

Roasting the plums gives them a deliciously juicy flavour,
and the cinnamon sugar adds a crisp coating.
Serve warm with crème fraîche, ice cream or custard.

Sugar plums

140g/5oz white granulated sugar
¼ tsp ground cinnamon
1 large egg white
12 red plums

Takes 25 minutes • Serves 4

1 Preheat the oven to 200°C/180°C fan/
gas 6. Mix the sugar and cinnamon in a
bowl. Whisk the egg white in a second bowl,
then roll the plums first in egg white, then the
cinnamon sugar until very well coated in a
sugary crust.
2 Space apart in a buttered baking dish,
then bake for 15 minutes or until the plums
are crusty, cooked through and starting to
be juicy. To test, poke the plums with a
cocktail stick; if it goes in easily, they are
ready to serve.

• Per serving 207 kcalories, protein 2g, carbohydrate
53g, fat none, saturated fat none, fibre 3g, sugar 53g,
salt 0.06g

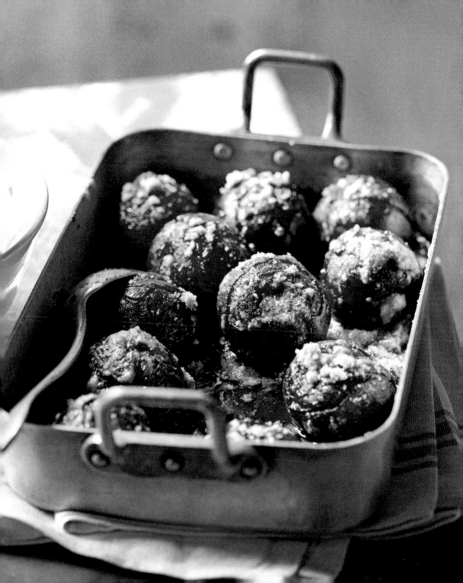

Index

bbcgoodfood.com

Great-value family food

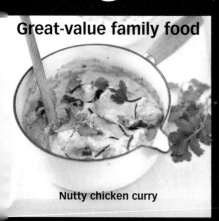

Nutty chicken curry

Easy weeknight suppers

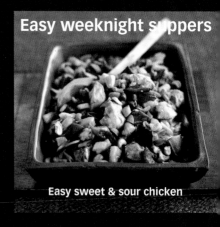

Easy sweet & sour chicken

Smart entertaining

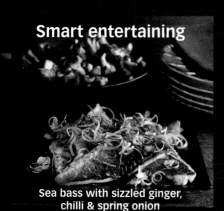

Sea bass with sizzled ginger, chilli & spring onion

Hundreds of desserts

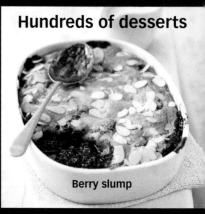

Berry slump

Over 6,000 recipes you can trust